WA 1323306 8

D1760340

APPLICATION OF MUSCLE/NERVE STIMULATION IN HEALTH AND DISEASE

Advances in Muscle Research

Volume 4

Series Editor

G.J.M. Stienen, *Vrije Universiteit, Amsterdam, The Netherlands*

Application of Muscle/Nerve Stimulation in Health and Disease

By

Gerta Vrbová
University College Medical School, London, UK

Olga Hudlicka
University of Birmingham Medical School, Birmingham, UK

and

Kristin Schaefer Centofanti
JKC Research Partnership, London, UK

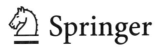 Springer

Gerta Vrbová
University College Medical School
London, UK

Kristin Schaefer Centofanti
JKC Research Partnership
London, UK

Olga Hudlicka
University of Birmingham Medical School
Birmingham, UK

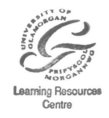

Learning Resources
Centre

13233068

ISBN: 978-1-4020-8232-0   e-ISBN: 978-1-4020-8233-7

Library of Congress Control Number: 2008922907

Printed on acid-free paper

9 8 7 6 5 4 3 2 1

springer.com

Acknowledgements

Without the help of Dr. Gillian Knight we would have been unable to complete the manuscript and cope with all the vagaries of our computers. Discussions with Dr. Milan Dimitrijevic pinpointed important points regarding the application of basic science to human physiology and treatment. We are grateful to Jorge Centofanti for his encouragement and help during the preparation of this manuscript. We are grateful to Ultratone for giving permission to reproduce the drawings in Chapter 4.

Introduction

The first evidence that electrical changes can cause muscles to contract was provided by Galvani (1791). Galvani's ideas about 'animal electricity' were explored during the 19th and 20th century when it was firmly established that 'electricity' is one of the most important mechanisms used for communication by the nervous system and muscle. These researches lead to the development of ever more sophisticated equipment that could either record the electrical changes in nerves and muscles, or elicit functional changes by electrically stimulating these structures. It was indeed the combination of these two methods that elucidated many of the basic principles about the function of the nervous system.

Following these exciting findings, it was discovered that electrical stimulation and the functions elicited by it also lead to long-term changes in the properties of nerves and particularly muscles. Recent findings help us to understand the mechanisms by which activity induced by electrical stimulation can influence mature, fully differentiated cells, in particular muscles, blood vessels and nerves. Electrically elicited activity determines the properties of muscle fibres by activating a sequence of signalling pathways that change the gene expression of the muscle. Thus, electrical activity graduated from a simple mechanism that is used to elicit muscle contraction, to a system that could induce permanent changes in muscles and modify most of its characteristic properties. These modifications induced by electrical stimulation are not random, but depend on the amount, as well as the precise pattern of activity. Thus certain types of activity will induce endurance, others increase force production. The regime of stimulation therefore needs to be tailored according to special requirements of the condition to be influenced.

The understanding of these stimulation-induced changes in muscle properties provides a powerful tool for manipulating, in a controlled manner, both normal and diseased muscles. Moreover, stimulation of damaged nerves and tissues seem to increase their potential for repair.

Thus the increased knowledge about the effects of electrical stimulation on various parts of our healthy or damaged body allows us to use stimulation as an efficient therapeutic tool.

Technical advances in the development of machines that allow efficient and easy methods of stimulation of human muscles and nerves allows us to exploit this knowledge for achieving adaptation of normal muscles to a desired type/shape, and to restore/maintain the properties of muscles that have deteriorated as a result of injury, disease, or other causes.

The present book summarizes the effects that long-term electrical stimulation has on muscle and its blood supply, and explains how these modifications can be applied to benefit healthy and sick people. It also provides a guide to be used to decide what type of stimulator is most suitable for particular conditions. Moreover it gives detailed instruction with precise illustrations about the most effective method for stimulating particular muscle groups.

Contents

to a muscle are excited there is a hierarchical order in which this is accomplished, i.e. first the small motoneurones are recruited (excited) and gradually the larger cells are called upon.[4,5] The significance of this arrangement for muscle function will be discussed later.

1.1.3   The Axon

The long extension of the motoneurone, its axon, is unique in that it leaves the CNS and navigates its way towards the muscle it innervates. The axons are covered by myelin that insulates the axon from the extracellular environment. However, not the entire length of the axon is insulated by the myelin. At regular intervals the axon is exposed and can communicate with the extracellular environment. The sites of this exposed part of the axon are called the nodes of Ranvier (see Fig. 1.2). The message along the axon is an electrical event. During rest, the membrane of the axon and the myelin sheath separates the environment inside the axon from that on the outside. When the axon is excited its membrane allows some movements of ions between the inside (intracellular) and outside (extracellular) of the axon. This movement of ions causes an electrical change, the action potential. The action potential is traveling along the axon by jumping from one node of Ranvier to the next. This allows it to travel much faster along the axon, and the rate at which it travels depends on the distance between successive nodes. The further apart they are, the faster is the conduction velocity of the action potential. The action potential is conducted along the whole axon and all its branches.[2,3]

On reaching the muscle, the axon divides into many branches. Each branch terminates on a muscle fibre and becomes a specialized structure called the ***axon terminal***. It is now that an interaction with the muscle fibre starts.

1.1.4   The Neuromuscular Junction

The motor nerve terminal has many specialized features. It contains a chemical, acetylcholine (ACh), that is packaged into tiny balloons (vesicles) and there is a special mechanism by which ACh is released when the electrical impulse reaches the terminal. When the electrical impulse invades the nerve terminal Ca^{2+} enters the nerve ending and this causes the vesicles containing ACh to fuse with the membrane of the nerve ending and the ACh to spill out. At the place of contact with the nerve terminal the muscle fibre develops a highly specialized structure, the motor endplate. Its most important feature is that it contains molecules that are able to combine with ACh: i.e. acetylcholine receptors (AChR) (Fig. 1.3). As soon as ACh is released from the nerve terminal it combines with the AChR and, as a result of this combination, produces an electrical change of the membrane of the muscle fibre at the endplate. Provided this change is great enough, it will be conducted

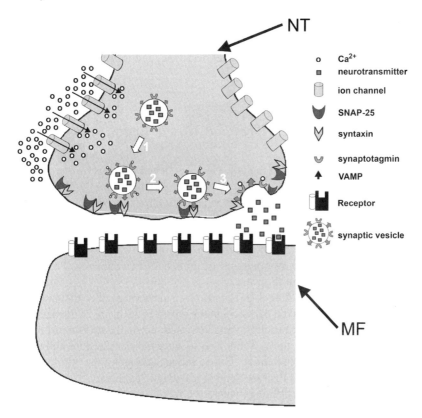

Fig. 1.3 A schematic representation of impulse transmission at the neuromuscular junction is shown. Ca^{2+} ions enter the nerve terminal (NT) through channels (yellow tubes). Their entry induces a sequence of molecular events. The Ca^{2+} ions combine with synaptotagmin on the surface of the synaptic vesicles that contain the transmitter acetylcholine (ACh). The synaptic vesicles are transported to the membrane of the NT where synaptosomal-associated protein of 25 kDa (SNAP-25) and syntaxin help the synaptic vesicles to fuse with the nerve terminal membrane and spill out their content. The ACh combines with the ACh receptor of the muscle fibre (MF) membrane. This opens up channels that cause the muscle fibre membrane to initiate an action potential along its entire surface. (Reproduced from http://www.bio.davidson.edu/courses/Bio111/Neurojunction. html with permission)

along the whole length of the muscle fibre and elicit a contraction. The ACh is rapidly destroyed by the enzyme cholinesterase, which is attached to the endplate. When the ACh is destroyed the electrical change of the membrane reverses to its normal state and the membrane is ready to respond again to ACh so that the muscle can be repeatedly activated.[2,3]

To summarize:

1. The motor nerve terminal is activated by an action potential.
2. Ca^{2+} enters the motor nerve terminal and causes the release of ACh.

3. ACh combines with the AChR of the muscle membrane and causes an electrical change.
4. ACh is destroyed by the enzyme cholinesterase, and a new impulse can excite the muscle.

1.1.5 Skeletal Muscle Fibres and Muscle Contraction

Skeletal muscles are structures that are usually attached to bones by tendons and by producing force can either move joints or help to stabilize them. Each muscle consists of numerous subunits or bundles called fascicles. These are surrounded by connective tissue and contain many individual muscle fibres (Fig. 1.4). Muscles specialize in the transformation of chemical energy into mechanical events, i.e. force production. Muscle fibres are cells specialized to carry out this task. Each muscle fibre is composed by a number of units called sarcomeres. These are the units that actually carry out the work.

Each individual muscle fibre is surrounded by a membrane called the sarcolemma. Like the membrane of the axon the sarcolemma separates the inside of the muscle fibre from the outside. When a muscle fibre is activated, normally at the neuromuscular junction, the sarcolemma allows some ions to enter the muscle fibre and this flow of ions initiates an action potential. This is propagated along the whole length of the muscle fibre. However, the sarcolemma has unique features; at regular intervals the sarcolemma has little openings where the membrane penetrates deep into the muscle cells and forms a system of tubes that are in close contact with the contractile machinery of the muscle cells (Fig. 1.5). These membranes carry the electrical impulse deep into the muscle fibre. Inside the muscle fibre the tubes communicate with structures (sarcoplasmic reticulum) that contain Ca^{2+}. When the muscle is electrically excited Ca^{2+} is released from these stores and it is this event that initiates movement. As soon as the electrical impulse terminates the Ca^{2+} is pumped back into its stores, so that at rest the levels of Ca^{2+} are very low and the muscle is relaxed.

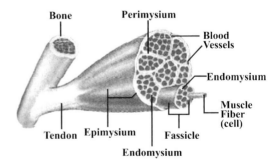

Fig. 1.4 Skeletal muscle with tendon attached. The picture shows a typical skeletal muscle with its tendon attached to a bone. The cut muscle illustrates its macroscopic structure, which includes the covering membranes of epimysium on the outside, of perimysium between muscle bundles (fascicles), and of endomysium around each muscle fibre, as well as the blood vessels that are within the muscle. (Reproduced from http://people.eku.edu/ritchisong/301notes3.htm with permission)

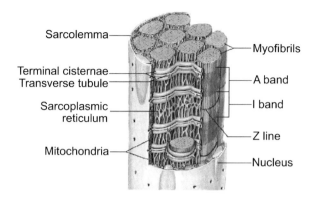

Fig. 1.5 Cross-section through a muscle fibre. A cross-section through a muscle fibre illustrates its contents: myofibrils, with their typical cross-striations due to the alignment of myosin (A band) and actin (I band), the Z line where the sarcomeres are attached to each other. In addition it shows the muscle membrane (sarcolemma), and structures connected to it, including the terminal cysternae and transverse tubules which allow the Ca^{2+} ions to reach the myofibrils. The sarcoplasmic reticulum and mitochondria are also shown; these structures are involved in removing the Ca^{2+} from the cytoplasm and keeping its concentration low during rest. (Reproduced from http://people.eku.edu/ritchisong/301notes3.htm with permission)

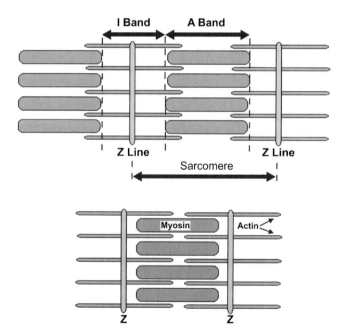

Fig. 1.6 Actin and myosin. Actin (green) and myosin (purple) are shown at rest (top panel), and during contraction (bottom panel). The shortening of the myofibres is clearly visible. (Reproduced from http://members.aol.com/Bio50/LecNotes/lecnot13.html with permission). To see the animated contraction go to http://people.eku.edu/ritchisong/301notes3.htm

Movement, i.e. force development, is accomplished by the interaction of two proteins, myosin and actin. These two proteins are arranged into regular units called sarcomeres. Figure 1.6 illustrates the arrangements of these proteins in a single sarcomere. At rest interaction between these proteins is prevented by another complex of proteins, troponins, but when the muscle fibre is electrically excited the troponin complex moves out of the way and allows the actin and myosin to slide against each other and produce force.

The sliding of the actin and myosin is the result of interactions between myosin heads (little flexible buds of the myosin) and the actin filaments. The myosin heads swivel and crawl along the actin, the sarcomere shortens and produces force (Fig. 1.7).

This event is allowed to occur when Ca^{2+} is released from internal stores and binds to troponin. Troponin has binding sites for Ca^{2+} ions and when Ca^{2+} binds to troponin its structure changes and it moves out of the way of the actin and myosin so that they are now free to slide against each other and produce force. As soon as the Ca^{2+} is removed from the binding site of troponin, the troponin and tropomysosin get back in place and prevent any interaction between the myosin and actin.

The energy needed for the mechanical work is provided by adenosine 5'-triphosphate (ATP). The enzyme myosin ATPase, splits this molecule and like an explosion energy is provided by this splitting of ATP. The energy is needed to detach the heads of the myosin molecules from the actin so that they are free to re-attach themselves again, continue to move along the actin and produce force.

Each muscle fibre contains many sarcomeres and they are connected to each other by proteins. In most mammalian muscles contraction of all sarcomeres occurs at the same time so that the whole muscle fibre develops force.

To summarize events that cause muscles to contract:

1. An electrical impulse travels along the muscle fibre membrane.
2. This electrical change causes the release of Ca^{2+} inside the muscle fibre.

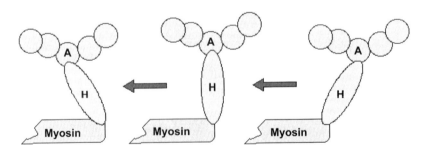

Fig. 1.7 The movement of myosin heads. The movement of the myosin heads (H) along the actin filament (A), which causes muscle contraction, is illustrated. (Reproduced from http://members. aol.com/Bio50/LecNotes/lecnot13.html with permission). To see the animated version of this event go to http://people.eku.edu/ritchisong/301notes3.htm

3. Ca^{2+} binds to troponin and temporarily displaces it from preventing the myosin and actin interactions.
4. Contact with actin initiates the myosin heads to swivel and form attachments to actin.
5. ATP breakdown provides the energy for detachment of the myosin head from actin so that another movement of the myosin head along the actin filament can take place.

1.1.6 *Muscle Function*

During a single impulse there is not enough time for the muscle to develop the force it is capable of producing. The contraction developed by the muscle in response to a single impulse is called a twitch, and usually develops only about one third of the force the muscle is capable of producing. Repeated stimulation of the muscle generates more force and these contractions are called tetanic contractions. Thus, a single impulse initiates a twitch contraction and repeated stimulation initiates tetanic contractions. The force generated by tetanic contractions, depends on the frequency of stimulation, i.e. intervals between successive impulses, and on the type of muscle in question. Some muscles contract and relax rapidly (fast muscles) and some slowly (slow muscles). Fast muscles need to be activated at higher frequencies to develop more force, slow muscles develop high forces already at lower rates of stimulation. Figure 1.8 illustrates this point. These facts show that force developed by a particular muscle depends on the frequency at which it is activated, and the type of muscle fibres it contains.[5]

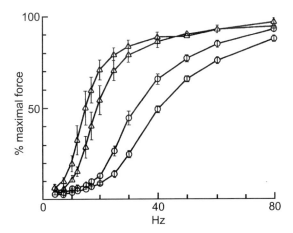

Fig. 1.8 Graph of maximum tetanic force against stimulation frequency. The percentage of maximum tetanic force developed by two slow (Δ) and two fast (O) motor units is plotted against the frequency of stimulation. The motor units are taken from a cat gastrocnemius muscle. (Reproduced from[5] with permission from Springer)

1.2   The Use of Muscles During Movement

The brief description of the components of the motor unit and some of its properties should provide us with an understanding of how muscles function during movement.

1.2.1   *Regulation of Force Production*

The first question we will consider is how the force of muscle contraction is regulated during voluntary movement.

To regulate force we use two main mechanisms[6]: (a) **Engaging more motor units to participate in the movement**. Since each individual muscle contains many motor units the strength of contraction of a muscle can be increased by activating a greater proportion of its motor units. In most muscles not all motor units are active during a particular movement and the force produced by a muscle can be increased by activating more motoneurones in the spinal cord and more motor units. An interesting feature of this regulation of force by motor unit recruitment is the fact that during movement the units that are activated first are the smallest units, which produce little force. The size of motoneurones that activate these units is relatively small and these motoneurones/motor units are activated during movements that require little force, such as posture. This regulation of force production by which the weakest units are activated first is referred to as the size principle (Fig. 1.9). As more force is required bigger motoneurones

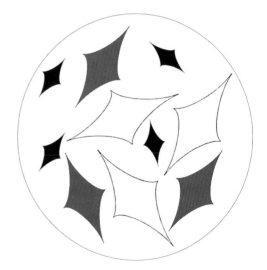

Fig. 1.9 Motoneurones. The different sizes and types of motoneurones within the spinal cord are schematically represented. The smallest most excitable are black, the intermediate are grey and the least excitable are white

are activated in the CNS and bigger increases in force are achieved by the active muscle. (b) **Increasing the frequency at which each motor unit is firing**. Due to properties of muscle fibres, a single stimulus allows the muscle to produce only about one third of the total force it is capable of producing. When the muscle is repeatedly activated the forces add up and the contraction is stronger. By repeated excitation the force developed by the muscle can be increased to reach its maximum at a certain frequency of stimulation. Different types of motor units require different frequencies of stimulation to allow them to produce more force (see Fig. 1.8). (c) **Finally, force production can be modified by a combination of (a) and (b)**.

1.2.2 *Differences Between Mammalian Muscles*

Skeletal muscles have a variety of functions during movement and at rest. Some muscles are highly specialized and used to help to support our joints and our posture. These are usually referred to as slow postural muscles and are anatomically situated around joints, or in the deeper layer of the musculature. Most muscle fibres in these muscles are used almost continuously and are adapted to this function. Other muscles are used for rapid movement and referred to as fast muscles.

The distinction into slow and fast muscles was first based on the different colour of the two types of muscles, a visibly different speed of contraction, and different resistance to fatigue.[7,8]

The majority of muscles are, however, mixed and perform various functions. Some parts are used to move joints, others to maintain posture. This multifunctional performance of our muscles is possible because they contain different motor units and each of these motor units is specialized for a particular function. The muscle fibres that different motor units use during movement are highly specialized and optimally suited for their function.

1.2.3 *Muscle Fibre Types*

When we examine muscle fibres in a skeletal muscle and reveal enzymes and proteins that individual muscle fibres contain, we find that the muscle fibres differ from each other. Figure 1.10 shows an example taken from a rabbit muscle that has been cut across its middle, and then a very thin section has been prepared and analysed for different enzymes that are important for the function of the muscle. In this particular picture, the enzyme that provides energy for the work the muscle is doing, the myosin ATPase, has been visualized. It is clear from this picture that some muscle fibres are darkly stained because they contain large amounts of the enzyme, some are light and some intermediate. How do we explain the presence of

Fig. 1.10 A cross-section of a rabbit extensor digitorum longus reacted for ATPase is shown to illustrate the different fibre types. The darkly stained fibres (type I) belong to slow motor units, the lighter ones (type IIA) to intermediate and the large white fibres (IIB) to fast motor units

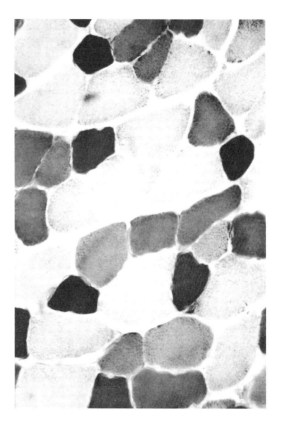

these different muscle fibre types within the same muscle? We have previously discussed that muscles are composed of individual motor units and that each motor unit functions independently. Strange as it seems, the muscle fibres belonging to different motor units are all mixed up within the muscle.

Nevertheless muscle fibres from the same motor unit are not different but are identical. Moreover, muscle fibres belonging to a particular motor unit are specialized according to the type of activity they are made to carry out during movement. Muscle fibres that belong to motor units that are active for long periods of time are specialized so as to allow them to work for long periods of time without fatigue and are called type I fibres. These muscle fibres contract and relax slowly and are therefore called slow muscle fibres. On the other hand muscle fibres of motor units that do not work very often fatigue rapidly and these are called type IIA and IIB fibres. Both type IIA and IIB muscle fibres contract and relax rapidly and are therefore called fast muscle fibres. Based on these physiological and biochemical differences, muscle fibres and motor units have been classified into three main types: fast fatiguable (IIB), fast fatigue resistant (IIA) and slow (I). This is illustrated in Figure 1.11.

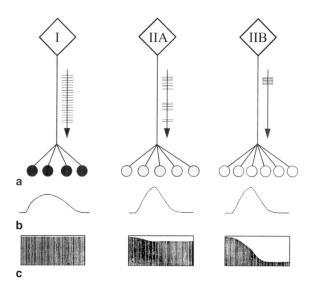

Fig. 1.11 The properties of three types of motor units in skeletal muscles are summarized in relation to their function. **(a)** The motoneurones are labelled I, IIA, and IIB according to the types of muscle fibres they innervate. The arrow with the horizontal lines across it alongside each 'axon' illustrates the type of activity transmitted by the motoneurone to the muscle fibres. The circles represent muscle fibres, black, type I, grey type IIA, white type IIB. **(b)** Single twitches of each type of motor unit are shown. **(c)** The decline of force with time in response to repeated tetanic contractions, i.e. muscle fatigue is illustrated. Type I muscle fibres do not fatigue, type IIB muscle fibres are slightly more fatiguable and type IIB muscle fibres fatigue rapidly. (Reproduced from[5] with permission from Springer)

1.3 Activity Determines Muscle Properties

The above description of the matching properties of muscle fibres to motoneurone activity already indicates the importance of motoneurone activity in determining the properties of muscle fibres it supplies.

1.3.1 Matching Properties of Muscles to Their Activity

Different skeletal muscles in the body contain various proportions of slow, intermediate and fast motor units, and this is related to their function in the body. Muscles involved predominantly in maintaining posture, or supporting a particular joint are composed predominantly of slow muscle fibres. These slow muscle fibres can maintain force for long periods of time without fatigue. Muscles used to move joints are composed predominantly of fast (IIA and IIB) muscle fibres that can produce force rapidly, but also fatigue more readily. Thus the motor system is perfectly adjusted to the type of activity it performs. How is this adjustment achieved?

The first indication that the motoneurone plays a leading role in determining the properties of muscle fibres it supplies was obtained in the 1960s. A group of researchers took advantage of findings that in some hind leg muscles particular types of muscle fibres were segregated. In the soleus muscle that stabilises the ankle joint, most of the fibres are slow contracting (Type I) and belong to motor units that are more or less continuously active, fatigue resistant and slow contracting. Another hindlimb muscle, tibialis anterior (TA) which controls the movement of the ankle joint and is active only when the foot is lifted off the ground, has motor units that are active intermittently and contains type IIA and IIB muscle fibres, which are fatiguable and fast contracting. So the soleus is a slow muscle and the TA is a fast muscle. The different patterns of activity imposed upon these two muscles and their different properties are illustrated in Fig. 1.12.

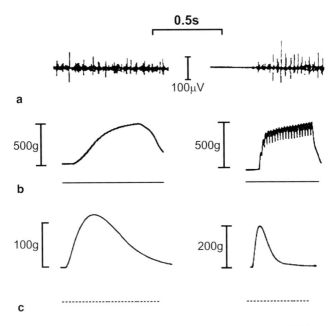

Fig. 1.12 Recordings from two rabbit hindlimb muscles: soleus (left) and tibialis anterior (right). (a) Electromyographic recordings from these muscles show continuous activity in the soleus muscle, whereas in the tibialis anterior muscle activity is only present when ankle movement was elicited by pinching the paw. (b) Records of tetanic contractions from the same muscles in response to stimulation at 40 Hz show that soleus muscles contracts slowly and the tetanic contraction is fused, whereas the tibialis anterior muscle contracts rapidly and the tetanus is not fused (see ripples). (c) Records of single twitches show that soleus (left) contracts and relaxes more rapidly then tibialis anterior (right). The intervals between the dots represents 10 ms. (Reproduced from[5] with permission from Springer)

Fig. 1.13 Cross-innervation of two rabbit hindlimb muscles: soleus and tibialis anterior. Recordings of contractions of the soleus muscle show that the slow time course of contraction becomes fast when the soleus receives the nerve that previously inner-vated the tibialis anterior muscle (a). The converse is true of the tibialis anterior muscle, which becomes slow contracting when it receives the soleus nerve (b). All recordings were carried out 3 months after cross-innervation

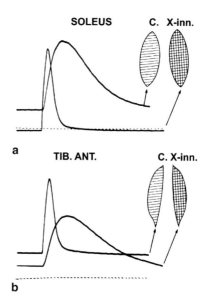

1.3.2 Changing Muscle Properties by Altering Their Innervation

When the nerves to these muscles with completely different properties were interchanged (X-inn) the slow soleus muscle which now was activated intermit-tently by the motoneurones that previously innervated the TA muscle became fast contracting (Fig. 1.13a) and the TA muscle became slow (Fig. 1.13b). Thus the nerve changed the contractile characteristics of these two hindlimb muscles.[9]

What tricks does the nerve use to achieve this? The simplest explanation is that it makes the slow soleus muscle work intermittently as though it is a TA muscle and the TA muscle work continuously as though it is a soleus muscle and that this change of the activity transforms the muscle from one type to another. If this was the case then it should be possible to achieve such changes without interfering with the nerve, but by imposing a novel pattern of activity on the muscle either by interfering with the control of movement or directly by electrical stimulation.

1.3.3 Changing Muscle Properties by Altering Their Activity

The soleus muscle of most mammals is a slow contracting (Fig. 1.14) postural muscle and is activated continuously during posture, which includes subtle changes of muscle length (Fig. 1.14a). These changes are mediated via sensors (muscle spindles) in the muscle and nerves that pass these signals to the motoneurones in the spinal cord.[3] When the muscle cannot be lengthened, or the signals from the special sense organs are interrupted, then the activity to the soleus motoneurones is reduced (Fig. 1.14b). After a few weeks of such reduced activity, the soleus muscles become to resemble fast muscles and no longer produces a sustained slow contraction (Fig. 1.14d). Thus without interrupting its nerve supply, soleus muscles can be changed when its activity is reduced. Reduction of activity can be achieved by temporarily stopping impulse traffic along the nerve by cutting the tendon, or by hindlimb suspension. All these manipulations produce changes in the slow soleus muscle that made it more similar to a fast muscle.

Moreover, if such a soleus muscle that had a reduced natural activity is electrically stimulated by a pattern of activity that resembles a normal soleus muscle, it will remain slow contracting and retain characteristics typical of a slow muscle[10] (Fig. 1.15 Top panel A and b) while activity typical of a fast muscle will not achieve this (Fig. 1.15 Bottom Panel A and B).

Can an originally fast muscle be converted into a slow one and acquire all the characteristic properties of a slow muscle? The answer is yes, provided the right type of activity is imposed on a fast muscle by electrical stimulation.[10] There is now overwhelming evidence that when fast mammalian skeletal muscles are activated electrically for several weeks by a pattern of activity that is normally typical of a slow muscle: i.e. it is more or less continuous, and the frequency is relatively slow, the fast muscles became to resemble slow muscles. They became slow contracting and fatigue resistant (Fig. 1.16).[10]

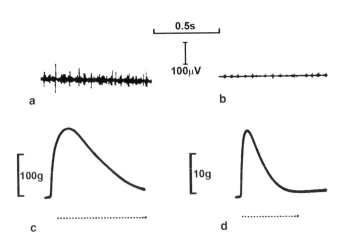

Fig. 1.14 Recordings from soleus muscles. Electromyographic record from (**a**) normal soleus, (**b**) after cutting its tendon, (**c**) twitch contraction from normal soleus, and (**d**) 1 month after cutting its tendon. (Reproduced from[5] with permission from Springer)

Fig. 1.15 Records of contractions taken from a control soleus muscle (top panel A and bottom panel A) and soleus muscles that had their tendons cut and were electrically stimulated at slow, 10Hz (top panel B) and fast 40Hz (bottom panel B). Note only the slow 10Hz stimulation preserved the slow contraction. (Reproduced from[10] with permission from Blackwell Publishers)

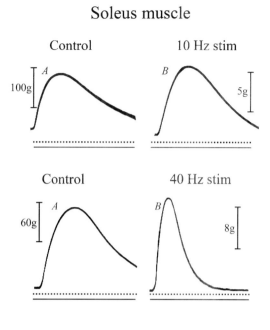

Fig. 1.16 Single twitches recorded from a control tibialis anterior (fast) and a tibialis anterior electrically stimulated for 3 weeks (slow) are superimposed. Note that the stimulated tibialis anterior became slow contracting. (Reproduced from[5] with permission from Springer)

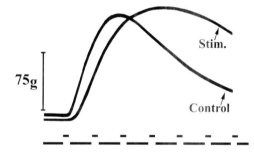

Several observations confirmed this finding and led to thorough investigations as to the molecular changes underlying this transformation. One example of such a change is the increase of oxidative enzymes in the fast TA muscles (Fig. 1.17).

Indeed, chronic low frequency stimulation has become an excellent model to study what (a) determines muscle properties, and (b) the different patterns of activity that do so. A series of investigations elucidated activity-induced changes in most components of skeletal muscle fibres and these have been described in several reviews[12] and are summarized in Fig. 1.18. Finally, so consistent and dramatic were the changes produced by a particular activity pattern employed during chronic stimulation that it lead to the hypothesis that activity is able to change gene expression in highly specialized cells such as muscle fibres.[13]

nerves, because the nerves inside the muscle are much more readily activated by electrical impulses then muscle fibres. It is possible that the muscle can only produce these adaptive changes when it is stimulated through its nerve, but if it were to be stimulated without the nerve it might not be able to respond to electrically induced activity and adapt.

If the nerve to a muscle is damaged then the motor axons in the muscle degenerate and disappear so that the muscle can no longer be excited by the nerve. Such a muscle is called a denervated muscle. Even though such a muscle can no longer be activated by its nerve it can be made to contract if the electrodes are placed directly onto the muscle and large currents are used to excite the muscle fibres themselves. Under these conditions only the muscle itself can be responsible for any stimulation-induced changes. When the adaptive potential of a denervated muscle was tested, it was found that just like a normal muscle its properties could be altered by electrical stimulation. The changes obtained depended on the type of activity imposed upon the muscle. When the denervated muscle was stimulated for long periods of time at low frequency it became a slow postural muscle, but when it was activated intermittently with burst at high frequencies it became a fast contracting muscle.[16] Thus the ability of the muscle to change its properties is inherent in the muscle itself and can occur without the nerve. However this situation arises only after injury to the nervous system or peripheral nerves.

1.5   Results on Human Muscles

Most of the results described here were those obtained from animal experiments. However there is now evidence that human muscles are responding to activity in a similar fashion as those of animals. Human leg muscles that have been inactive for long periods of time become more fatiguable and resemble fast muscles.[17] Inactivity has many other deleterious effects on human muscles, such as loss of weight and reduced ability to produce force. These changes are a great disadvantage in many situations where restoration of function is attempted, and it is therefore of great importance to reverse or prevent them. This indeed can be achieved by electrical stimulation of the inactive muscles. In several studies on patients that had inactive muscles, either due to injury or bed rest, it was shown that most inactivity induced deterioration of the muscles can be reversed by appropriate electrical stimulation.

In a recent study on patients with spinal cord injury it was shown that even if the muscles lost their innervation their function could be restored by electrical stimulation.[18]

The possibility of restoring inactivity-induced changes in human muscles is extremely important in many situations discussed in another chapter of this book.

1.6   Comparison of Electrical Stimulation to Exercise

Muscle activity induced by electrical stimulation is in many respects unnatural and has often been viewed with some reservation. Two fundamental differences exist between voluntary or reflexly elicited contractions and those induced by electrical stimulation of muscle. During voluntary or reflex movements motor units are activated asynchronously and a strict hierarchical order of recruitment is always maintained. During this hierarchical recruitment of motor units the smallest motor units are activated first followed by contractions of larger units. Therefore during voluntary movement the largest motor units are least active and are used only during maximal effort. When electrical stimulation of the muscle is used to activate the muscles this order of recruitment is cancelled; indeed due to the biophysical properties of the axons that innervate the muscle the largest motor units are activated preferentially and therefore the parts of the muscle that are usually used rarely are active most frequently. However during electrical stimulation it is the motor units that are normally least active that experience the biggest increase in their use and consequently the biggest change in their characteristic properties. Thus electrical stimulation by bypassing the hierarchical order of recruitment, indeed by reversing it, is able to activate those motor units and muscle fibres that are only activated during most strenuous exercise. It can therefore exploit the adaptive potential of muscles more efficiently then exercise and maintain much higher levels of activity over time then exercise. This enhanced activity is restricted to specific target muscles and is unlikely to have unwanted systemic effects. Finally, high amounts of activity can be imposed on a muscle from the beginning, since the CNS, cardiovascular and other systems will not interfere or limit the amount of activity carried out by the muscle, as is the case during exercise.[12]

On the other hand, there are several functions that electrical stimulation of individual muscle groups cannot accomplish and that are unique to exercise induced activity. During exercise-induced activity coordinated movement is carried out and it is therefore likely that the individual's skills in carrying out movement of this kind will improve. Thus, while exercise can improve coordination, electrical stimulation is unlikely to do so. In addition the flexibility of joints and lengthening of muscles can be improved by exercise but not by electrical stimulation. Particular exercise regimes such as Pilates and yoga are particularly effective in achieving these goals.

Improvement of the cardiovascular system is also more easily achieved by exercise. Nevertheless, it can be argued that having muscles that are less fatiguable then usual, an advantage that is readily achieved by electrical stimulation, enables the individual to exercise more efficiently and achieve all the goals regarding fitness more readily and in a shorter time.

Acknowledgement   I am grateful to my colleagues who helped me over the years to improve my understanding of the subject discussed in this chapter. I would like to give special thanks to Prof. G. Burnstock for creating the conditions that enabled me to write this chapter, and above all to Dr. Gillian E. Knight without whose help I could not have completed this task.

References

1. C. Sherrington, The correlation of reflexes and the principle of common final path, *Brit. Ass.* **74**:728–741 (1939).
2. B. Katz, *Nerve Muscle and Synapse* (McGraw-Hill, New York, 1966).
3. E. R. Kandel, J. H. Schwartz, and T. M. Jessel, *Principles of Neural Science* (McGraw-Hill, New York, 2000).
4. E. Henneman, G. Somjen, and D. O. Carpenter, Functional significance of cell size in spinal motoneurones, *J. Neurophysiol.* **28**:560–580 (1965).
5. G. Vrbová, T. Gordon, and R. Jones, *Nerve-Muscle Interaction* (Chapman & Hall, London, 1995).
6. H. S. Milner-Brown, and R. B. Stein, The relation between the surface electromyogram and muscle force, *J. Physiol.* **246**:549–569 (1975).
7. L. Ranvier, De quelques faits relatifa à l'histologie et à la physiologie des muscles striés, *Arch. Physiol. Norm. Path.* **6**:1–15 (1874).
8. D. Denny-Brown, On the nature of postural reflexes, *Proc. Roy. Soc. (Biol.)* **104**:252–301 (1929).
9. A. J. Buller, J. C. Eccles, and R. M. Eccles, Interactions between motoneurones and muscles in respect of the characteristic speeds of their responses, *J. Physiol.* **150**:417–439 (1960).
10. S. Salmons, and G. Vrbová, The influence of activity on some contractile characteristics of mammalian fast and slow muscles, *J. Physiol.* **201**:535–549 (1969).
11. D. Pette, M. E. Smith, H. W. Staudte, and G. Vrbová, Effects of long-term electrical stimulation on some contractile and metabolic characteristics of fast rabbit muscle, *Pflüger's Arch.* **338**:257–272 (1973).
12. D. Pette, and G. Vrbová, What does chronic electrical stimulation teach us about muscle plasticity? *Muscle Nerve* **22**:666–677 (1999).
13. E. R. Chin, E. N. Olson, J. A. Richardson, Q. Yano, C. Humphries, J. M. Shelton, H. Wu, W. G. Zhu, R. Basselduby, and R. S. Williams, A calcineurin-dependent transcriptional pathway controls skeletal muscle fibre type, *Gene Devel.* **12**:2499–2509 (1998).
14. G. Vrbová, The effect of motoneurone activity on the speed of contraction of striated muscle, *J. Physiol.* **169**:513–526 (1963).
15. J. Tothova, B. Blaauw, G. Pallafacchina, R. Rudolf, C. Argentini, C. Reggiani, S. Schiaffino, NFATc1 nucleocytoplasmic shuffling is controlled by nerve activity in skeletal muscle, *J. Cell. Sci.* **119**:1604–1611 (2006).
16. A. Windisch, K. Gundersen, M. J. Szabolcs, H. Gruber, and T. Lomo, Fast to slow transformation of denervated and electrically stimulated rat muscle, *J. Physiol.* **510**:623–632 (1998).
17. A. J. R. Lenman, F. M. Tulley, G. Vrbová, M. R. Dimitrijevic, and J. A. Towle, Muscle fatigue in some neurological disorders, *Muscle Nerve* **12**:938–942 (1989).
18. H. Kern, K. Rossini, U. Carraro, W. Mayr, M. Vogelauer, U. Hoelwarth, and C. Hofer, Muscle biopsies show that FES of denervated muscles reverses human muscle degeneration from permanent spinal motorneuron lesion, *J. Rehabil. Res. Dev.* **42**:43–53 (2005).

Chapter 2
Cardiovascular System: Changes with Exercise Training and Muscle Stimulation

Olga Hudlicka

Abstract This chapter explains the function of the heart, regulation of blood pressure and blood flow and the importance of endothelial vessel lining in the normal adult organism. It also shows the importance of capillary supply in the function of skeletal and heart muscle and the effect of training and skeletal muscle electrical stimulation on these parameters. Many of these functions are changed in aging, hypertension, heart failure, peripheral vascular diseases, muscle immobilisation and denervation, spinal cord injuries and healing wounds. The beneficial effect of exercise training and muscle stimulation on the cardiovascular system in these diseased states are explained and compared.

Keywords Heart, blood pressure, large blood vessels, arterioles, capillaries, shear stress, endothelial function and dysfunction, aging, hypertension, heart failure, stroke, peripheral vascular diseases, oedema, muscle atrophy, spinal cord injuries, wounds

2.1 Function of the Cardiovascular System in the Normal Adult

2.1.1 Heart and Peripheral Circulation

The heart in an adult 70 kg heavy man pumps about 5–5.5 litres blood per minute from the left ventricle to the body via the largest vessel, the aorta. The same amount goes from the right ventricle through another large vessel, the pulmonary artery, to the lungs where the blood takes in oxygen from the air and releases carbon dioxide that had been carried from different tissues as a waste product of tissue metabolism. The oxygenated blood is distributed through a system of large and smaller vessels to all organs in the body. Blood to the head including the brain, goes through the carotid arteries, to the heart via the coronary and to the kidneys via renal arteries, to the arms via brachial and to the legs via femoral arteries. Blood flow through the heart and the vessels in explained in Fig. 2.1.

Department of Physiology, University of Birmingham Medical School, Birmingham B15 2TT UK

G. Vrbová et al., *Application of Muscle/Nerve Stimulation in Health and Disease*,   23
© Springer Science + Business Media B.V. 2008

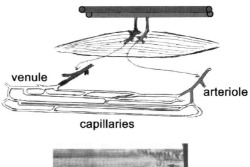

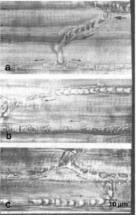

Fig. 2.3 Vascular supply and microcirculation in skeletal muscle. Top: A feed artery (sometimes one, more frequently more than one) is branching from a larger artery and after entering the muscle divides into numerous arterioles. These are eventually divided into numerous capillaries with interconnections and blood then enters a venule, larger venules and vein. (Modified according to[5].) Bottom. Real picture of capillary flow in skeletal muscle as observed under the microscope (a) arrow shows flow of the red blood cells from a small arteriole into two capillaries (b) flow in a capillary with many (top) and fewer (bottom) red blood cells (c) flow from capillaries into a venule. Note that red blood cells have different shape depending on their number and interval in individual capillaries. (From[6] with permission of Elsevier.)

2.3 Exercise and Electrical Stimulation Can Change Muscle Metabolism, Performance, Capillary Supply and Blood Flow

2.3.1 Changes in the Cardiovascular System During Acute Exercise

Skeletal muscles are the main tissues activated during exercise. To meet their demand for blood flow, cardiac output has to increase. This increase (by about 20% during mild, and up to 300% during strenuous exercise) varies with the number of

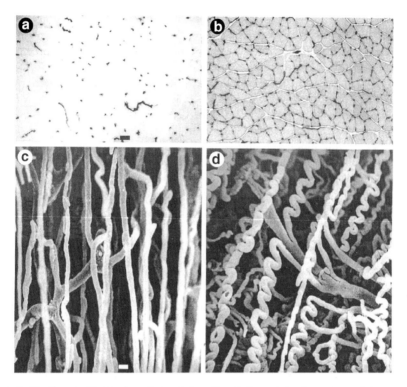

Fig. 2.4 Capillary bed in fast (**a** and **c**) and slow (**b** and **d**) rat skeletal muscles. a & b are cross sections of a fast (extensor digitorum longus, EDL; Fig. 2.4a) and slow soleus (Fig. 2.4b) muscle with staining depicting capillaries as black dots. Note that EDL has fewer capillaries than soleus. c & d are casts of the vascular bed in EDL (and soleus). The vessels were injected via the aorta with polymer. The muscles were taken 1 h later and muscle tissue was digested overnight. The casts were then coated with platinum and examined using the scanning electron microscope (from[3])

contracting muscles and the intensity of contraction. It is enabled by increase in stroke volume and in heart rate. However, in order to allow enough time for the blood to be brought back to the heart and to fill the heart ventricles adequately, the heart rate should not increase more than 180 beats per minute. If it exceeds this value, the duration of diastole will be too short for the heart ventricles to fill with enough blood so that the amount expelled during the following contraction (systole) will be too small and cardiac output would not increase enough. As the volume of blood ejected by each heart beat is limited, the total cardiac output is redistributed to meet the need of more active organs. Thus, during strenuous exercise over 70% of the total cardiac output is going to the muscles, and only 11% to the kidneys and the abdominal organs, 4.3% to the heart as well as to the brain, even if in absolute value the brain receives the same amount of blood as under resting conditions and the heart about three time more.

While the increase in muscle blood flow during muscle contractions is initiated by many factors, the increase in the cardiac output and its redistribution is
due mainly to the higher activity of the nerves which augment the force of the
heart contraction and increase heart rate. They also constrict vessels to the organs
not involved in exercise such as kidneys and liver. These nerves are activated
partly by the higher nerve centres in the brain, partly by a set of nerve fibres
turned on by muscle movements and changes in muscle metabolism occurring
with skeletal muscle contraction. The sum of these nervous activities results in an
increase in systolic blood pressure while diastolic pressure remains more or less
constant.[7]

It is still not quite clear what initiates the increase in muscle blood flow. It is
likely to be the result of many factors acting in coordination. The primary force
causing blood to flow through vessels is the difference in pressures between the
arterial and venous part of the vascular bed. The first few muscle contractions
squeeze blood out of the veins and the pressure there lowers. The pressure difference between arteries and veins thus increases and initiates the increase in flow.
Contracting muscles release a number of various metabolites that cause relaxation
of the smooth muscle cells in arterioles. This enables more blood to enter the
capillaries and therefore there are many more red blood cells in each capillary than

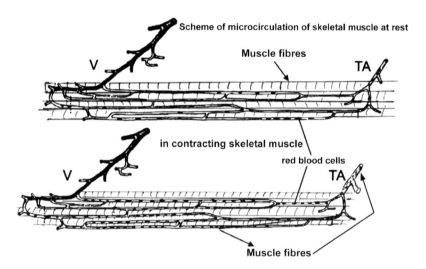

Fig. 2.5 Scheme of muscle microcirculation at rest and during isometric contraction. TA =
terminal arteriole, V = collecting venule. Red blood cells (RBC) are depicted as black dots.
Capillaries in a resting muscle have fewer RBC and some capillaries have none, but are still visible under the microscope. During contractions, the terminal arteriole is dilated (has a larger
diameter than at rest) and almost all capillaries are filled with RBC which also move much faster
that at rest. Various metabolites released from contracting muscle fibres act on smooth muscle
cells in the terminal arteriole and dilate it. They also act on capillary endothelium (arrows from
muscle fibre to terminal arteriole (TA) and to a capillary. This causes perfusion of more capillaries
with red blood cells and their increased velocity. Capillary endothelium can send signals towards
terminal arteriole and up to the other arterioles and feed artery (ascending dilatation)

at rest. Relaxation of smooth muscle cells in the smallest arterioles spreads towards the larger arterioles and to the feed arteries via the endothelium and allows a great increase in the inflow to the whole muscle (Fig. 2.5).

The increased flow causes an increased friction of blood against the endothelial lining of the vessel wall (called shear stress) and this force triggers a release of various substances from the endothelial cells that help to sustain the dilatation[8] (Fig. 2.6).

Dilatation of arterioles allows a greater amount of blood to enter capillaries and thus to improve the delivery of oxygen and nutrients, and removal of metabolites, such as lactic acid. The distribution of red blood cells in capillaries in resting muscles is not homogeneous: some have very large gaps between individual cells while others have cells tightly packed and very few capillaries have only plasma without red blood cells (see Fig. 2.4). However, this distribution changes in time and space, and the red blood cells also move, in some capillaries fast, in others slowly. This inhomogeneity of perfusion, as it is called, changes dramatically in contracting muscles: with increasing frequency and intensity of contractions more and more capillaries have red cells with smaller gaps between cells and the velocity of movement of individual cells increases. Consequently the distance from red blood cells to the centre of any muscle fibre is smaller and the supply of oxygen is better. As the velocity of capillary flow during muscle contractions increases, the

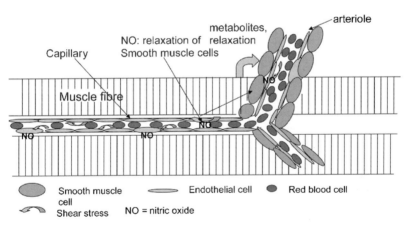

Fig. 2.6 Interaction of capillary shear stress, metabolites released from muscle fibres and endothelial cells and relaxation and contraction of smooth muscle cells. Vessels dilate when smooth muscle cells in their walls relax and constrict when they contract. Contraction of the smooth muscle cells can be elicited by the action of nerves or hormones (adrenalin, noradrenalin, angiotensin and others). Relaxation is due to metabolites released from skeletal muscle fibres during contractions, and also from muscle fibres undergoing atrophy. It can also be induced by various substances released from endothelial cells exposed to shear stress such as nitric oxide (NO). Inadequate release of NO under various conditions (aging, hypertension, heart failure, peripheral vascular diseases etc) causes inadequate relaxation of the smooth muscle cells and thus lack of dilatation and increased flow during muscle contraction or after short term limitation of blood flow (reactive hyperaemia)

exchange of fluid and the lymph flow is also higher and this is very important in the treatment of various conditions, as we will discuss later.

Blood flow during isometric contraction, during which the muscle does not change length but develops force without shortening, increases usually much less than during contractions when the length of the muscle changes. As the force of isometric contraction increases, blood flow actually stops as the pressure, developed by the force of muscle contraction is greater than the arterial pressure.

The increase in flow varies with muscle type and with the type, duration and intensity of exercise. Different types of activity increase blood flow in different types of muscles. During exhaustive exercise, blood flow increases in fast contracting or mixed muscles. During sprinting it rises only in fast contracting muscles and exercise of moderate intensity and prolonged duration enhances it in muscles or their parts composed of highly oxidative fibres.[9] The absolute increase during mild contractions in muscles composed of slow contracting muscle fibres with high oxidative metabolism is relatively small as their resting flow is several times higher than in the fast contracting muscles.

2.3.2 The Effect of Endurance Training

Endurance exercise training results in increased cardiac stroke volume, mainly due to increased contractility of the heart muscle. This is facilitated by increased venous return (that is more blood entering the heart during each diastole due to muscle movements and changes in respiration). Both help to propel the blood back to the heart and increase the filling of the ventricles – an important factor in increasing the force of cardiac muscle contraction. In the long-term, this leads to enlargement of individual muscle cells in the heart and increased heart weight – in other words heart hypertrophy. At the same time the increased force of heart muscle contractions activates some growth factors which are important in stimulating growth of capillaries and larger vessels supplying the heart so that the nutrition of the enlarged heart is well maintained. As the stroke volume increases, the need to increase cardiac output by increasing heart rate diminishes, and in well trained athletes the resting heart rate is actually considerably lower (sometimes as low as 40 beat per minute) than in untrained people. In spite of increased stroke volume blood pressure is not higher mainly because the vessels in working muscles dilate and the resistance to flow is diminished. In the end, blood pressure in trained athletes is slightly lower than in untrained people.[10]

Training leads to many changes in the whole organism, but they first appear in skeletal muscles. The capacity to extract oxygen from blood is much higher in endurance trained athletes. Consequently, the need to increase blood flow for the same amount of exercise is smaller, provided the exercise is performed at submaximal levels. At rest muscle blood flow is slightly lower than in untrained people. With maximal work load muscle blood flow increases more in endurance trained people than in control subjects; however the increase is similar to controls in sprinters. Experimental work that allowed measurements of flow in muscles with different muscle fibre composition showed that sprint training resulted in increased flow in fast contracting muscles with glycolytic metabolism with no change in slow contracting highly oxidative muscles while the reverse was true for endurance training (Fig. 2.7). Strength training does not alter muscle blood flow either at rest or during contractions. Due to reduced activity of sympathetic nerves in trained subjects, the reduction of blood flow in non-working organs such as the liver is less than in untrained people.

Training leads to extensive changes in the structure of the vascular bed. Different types of training cause growth of new capillaries depending of the type of muscle, or muscle fibres that are involved. Endurance training increases capillary supply in muscles composed of mainly oxidative fibres. In fast contracting muscles with glycolytic (predominantly anaerobic) metabolism capillary supply increases with sprint training (Fig. 2.7) whilst strength training has little effect. Endurance training also increases the total capillary transport capacity for water and solutes. The number of small vessels branching into capillaries and arterioles increases with

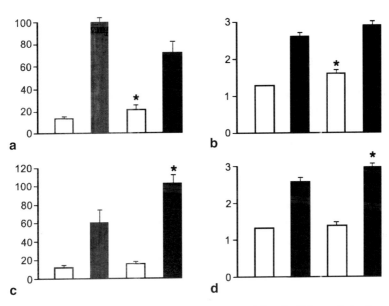

Fig. 2.7 The effect of training on capillary supply and blood flow in different skeletal muscles. High intensity sprint training (top panels) and low intensity endurance training (bottom panels) affect differently muscle blood flow ml/100g/min[-1] (a, c) and capillary supply (c/f ratio, b, d) in muscles with predominantly glycolytic (empty columns) and oxidative (black columns) muscle fibres. Blood flow and capillary supply is always higher in oxidative than glycolytic muscles and is not altered by sprint (top) training. It is increased by endurance training (bottom): the height of the black columns is higher after training than before and this is marked by asterisks. In contrast, endurance training does not affect either blood flow or capillary supply in glycolytic muscles (the height of the white columns does not change) but sprint training increases both as shown by the higher white columns in the top part of the figure, * denotes the differences. First 2 columns of each graph represent values before training and the second 2 columns of each graph represent values after training. (Modified according to[11].)

endurance training but is not altered by sprint training. Endurance training also increases the diameter of arterioles and feed arteries. This enables the increase in muscle blood flow to muscle groups involved in any particular type of training during maximal performance.[12]

In contrast to endurance training, training for strength, so called resistance training, increases blood pressure and cardiac output and leads to heart hypertrophy. Although the diameter of the arteries supplying the bulk of trained muscles (brachial artery in strength training of arms, femoral artery in strength training of leg muscles) increases, the findings on the changes in capillary supply are rather controversial and mostly agree on only very modest, if any, increase.

Growth of new vessels resulting from increased muscle activity is initiated by increased blood flow and some growth factors. As mentioned above, blood flow in skeletal muscles increases with each contraction. This is due to a number of mainly metabolic factors which produce dilatation of the smallest arterioles that spreads towards large vessels. Higher blood flow and higher velocity of red blood cell movement causes a greater friction between the blood and the vessel walls (shear stress) and, in turn, release of substances like NO from the endothelium. This, together with some growth factors, starts growth of the smallest vessels, capillaries.[12] Gradually, some of the capillaries are changed into arterioles and the whole vascular bed in trained muscles expands. Increased blood flow and the resulting release of NO causes enlargement (wider diameters) even in larger vessels like the aorta, brachial and femoral arteries. Growth of capillaries as well as arterioles occurs not only in skeletal muscles, but also in the hearts of trained animals. Indeed, the hearts of so called athletic animals like hares, greyhounds or racing horses have a much higher capillary supply than rabbits, other types of dogs or normal horses.[12] Training improves endothelial function[13] by increasing production of NO in endothelial cells and in muscle fibres. (NO is an important factor involved in the relaxation of the vascular smooth muscle cells as well as in capillary growth.) This is one of the reasons why training is essential in the maintenance of the normal vessel reactivity under various pathological circumstances as it will be shown in the following chapters.

2.3.3   Changes in the Circulation in Skeletal Muscles Induced by Electrical Stimulation

Muscle activity can be increased not only by training, but also by electrical stimulation of individual muscle groups. This involves activation of all muscle fibres within the stimulated muscles, as explained in Chapter 1. However, stimulation is usually performed only in a limited number of muscles or muscle groups involving a much smaller muscle mass than training, particularly endurance training. Consequently, the general changes in the cardiovascular system, such as cardiac output or blood pressure, are much smaller than those occurring with training. Nevertheless, some alterations have been observed in vessels in organs remote from the stimulated muscles. Although stimulation has been applied to different muscle groups, the knowledge of its effect on the vascular system is based almost predominantly on observations in leg muscles (or hind limbs in animals).

Experimental studies have shown that after low frequency electrical stimulation capillaries begin to grow very early (after only 2 days) prior to most modifications of muscle metabolism. This is due to a combination of increased activation of growth factors and substances released from vessel endothelium by increased shear stress (Fig. 2.6) which increases with every single muscle contraction.[14] The number of capillaries and their total area increases gradually with time reaching a plateau after approximately 1 month[15] and persists for about 6 weeks after the termination of stimulation. New capillaries first appear around the muscle fibres with glycolytic (anaerobic) metabolism which stimulation activates preferentially to other fibres (see Chapter 1). This is different from endurance exercise which recruits predominantly oxidative muscle fibres with capillary growth appearing first around these fibres. However with continuous stimulation capillaries appear everywhere so the capillary network is very dense and becomes homogeneously distributed (Fig. 2.8).

Capillaries also become more tortuous (Fig. 2.9).

This, as well as their increased numbers, increases their surface area available for exchange of nutrients, water and oxygen and thus allow improvement of muscle

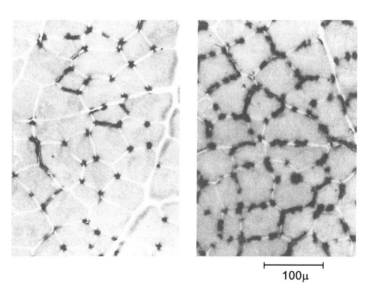

100μ

Fig. 2.8 The effect of electrical stimulation of fast muscles (extensor digitorum longus and tibialis anterior). Cross section of a rat extensor digitorum longus that had been stimulated at a frequency naturally occurring in nerves supplying slow muscle (10 impulses per second, for 8 h per day) for 7 days (right) and of a control muscle (left). The capillaries are represented as black dots. Compare with Fig. 2.4

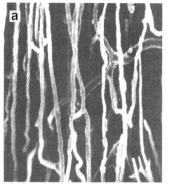 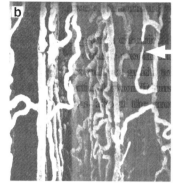

CONTROL MUSCLE	MUSCLE STIMULATED AT 10 Hz
(− 10μm)	CONTINUOUSLY 8h/DAY FOR 7 DAYS

Fig. 2.9 Casts of the microvasculature from control and electrically stimulated muscles. The technique is described in the legend to Fig. 2.4. Capillaries in the stimulated muscle are more numerous and more tortuous. It is possible to see a newly grown capillary as a sprout (arrow). (From[16] with kind permission of Springer Science and Business Media.)

metabolism. Capillary growth in stimulated muscles is followed by growth of arterioles and slightly higher maximal muscle blood flow (Fig. 2.10).

Electrical stimulation in patients increased blood flow and transport through capillaries more than endurance training.[17] It also increased the venous pump[18] (the amount of blood leaving the muscles during contractions) and improved lymph flow thus reducing the possibility of swelling (oedema formation).[19] Stimulation reduces the effect of vasoconstrictor nerves and substances causing constriction of vessels, such as noradrenalin, and improves the capacity of the endothelial cells to generate NO and thus their vasodilatation (Fig. 2.10). All these changes enhance the delivery of oxygen and nutrients to muscle cells and removal of waste products and thus improve muscles resistance to fatigue. Improved muscle performance and capillary growth following electrical stimulation were also described in human muscles.[20]

Stimulation at low frequencies (10 Hz) is most effective, but intermittent stimulation at higher frequencies (e.g. 40 Hz) leads to an increase in the number of capillaries similar to that achieved by low frequency stimulation, although the onset of the growth is delayed. Moreover, capillary and arteriolar growth can also be elicited by long-term administration of drugs that produce vasodilatation as the most important factor initiating vessel growth induced by electrical stimulation is increased blood flow.

Changes in the vasculature in stimulated muscles occur much earlier than those induced by exercise training and are more homogeneous over the whole muscle. Moreover, some of them, like the increase in the filtration capacity (transport of substances outside capillaries in the close contact with muscle fibres) which is an indicator of the total capillary surface area, were greater when induced by short term (4 weeks) electrical stimulation than by long term (several years) endurance training.[17]

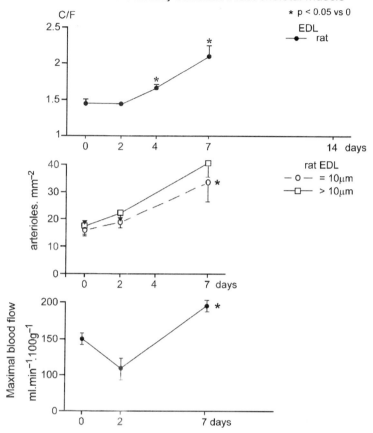

Fig. 2.10 Changes in the vascular bed in stimulated rat muscles. The number of capillaries expressed as capillary:muscle fibre ratio – top) gradually increases and is about 70% higher after 7 days of low-frequency stimulation than in control muscles (day 0). The number of small (=10μm) and larger (>10μm) arterioles (middle part) is increased to a similar extent. Total muscle blood flow (bottom) in contracting muscles is higher

2.4 Changes in the Cardiovascular System in Disease

2.4.1 Aging

The whole cardiovascular system changes with increasing age. The size of the cells in the heart increases and so does the thickness of the left ventricular wall. There is an increased proportion of collagen, a substance which produces stiffness of the ventricular wall and consequently both ventricular filling and emptying is more sluggish. The capacity of the cardiac pump is thus lower. Although heart rate is similar in old and young people, it does increase much less in the former during exercise, and so does cardiac output. Blood pressure increases with advancing age because the elasticity of the large vessels is lower and they cannot expand to accommodate the volume of blood ejected by the heart. The gradual development of arteriosclerosis with increasing age also contributes to the diminished elasticity of the large vessels. The deteriorated endothelial function (called endothelial dysfunction), characterised by impaired ability of endothelial cells which form the vessel lining to generate various substances important in the regulation of the vessel diameter, changes in permeability and ability to prevent blood clotting, plays a part in the impaired vasodilatation and in an increased tendency for thrombus formation and vessel occlusion. The higher activity of the vasoconstrictor nerves in old age results in an elevated resistance to blood flow and thus leads to higher blood pressure.[21]

Blood flow in skeletal muscles during exercise is lower in the arms, but remains unchanged in the legs. This is explained by the fact that leg muscles are more active than those in the arms in the course of the life span, their vessels have better blood flow and thus maintain better their endothelial cell function. Impaired endothelial function occurs not only in larger vessels such as brachial and femoral artery, but also in vessels in skeletal muscles and skin. The increased resistance to flow in these vessels is due to a diminished capacity to release NO and other substances contributing to vessel dilatation but also to the fact that elevated activity of vasoconstrictor nerves blunts the dilatation caused by various metabolites. The bulk of muscle tissue decreases between the third and eighth decade and represents a loss of 30–40% of the proportion of fibres with anaerobic metabolism. The number of capillaries supplying these fibres decreases while muscle fibres with high oxidative metabolism maintain their capillary supply. The number of arterioles also decreases and the capacity of larger vessels distant from capillaries and small arterioles (feed arteries) to dilate is diminished. All these changes result in a smaller increase in muscle blood flow during exercise. As the muscle ability to extract oxygen from blood is also lower in old age, muscles fatigue more easily.

Although old age affects circulation also in the skin this change is smaller than in skeletal muscle and temporary stoppage of flow is followed by a smaller increase in old than in young individuals. This may cause problems in elderly patients with restricted movements when their skin is exposed to prolonged pressure. Therefore bed-ridden elderly patients suffer from bed sores.

Some of these changes due to age can be reduced by exercise. Endurance training decreases systolic blood pressure, reduces the stiffness of the arteries and increases capillary supply in trained muscles in old animals as well as in patients. The decreased blood flow in old age is found mainly in highly oxidative muscles and training improves muscle oxidative metabolism. Training also improves the impairment of endothelial function in the elderly. It enhances the ability of vessels to dilate and decreases their tendency to thrombus formation. Well trained athletes have fewer atherosclerotic plaques in large arteries.[22]

Long-term low frequency electrical stimulation changes the pattern of fibre types in a similar degree in old as in young subjects, but little is known about its effect on the cardiovascular system. As with young subjects, hardly any improvements can be expected in the performance of the heart or blood pressure, as stimulation involves usually only small muscle groups. There are no data on muscle blood flow, but skin blood flow was improved by stimulation in elderly patients. Capillary supply in stimulated muscles increased to a similar degree in old as in young or middle aged animals. However, as stimulation induces capillary growth preferentially in the vicinity of glycolytic fibres where the capillary density decreases with old age, chronic electrical stimulation could be of a greater benefit than endurance exercise in old age.

2.4.2 Hypertension

High blood pressure, or hypertension, has many different causes, but the most important alterations in the cardiovascular system are similar. The large arteries like the aorta are more rigid due to the increased content of collagen. Smaller arteries in hypertensive animals or human beings have usually more smooth muscle cells and are narrower thus impeding blood flow. Consequently, the heart works against a greater resistance and the size of its cells as well as the whole cardiac muscle mass increases. This could improve the force of contraction. However, as the capillaries supplying the cardiac muscle do not grow, the muscle cells in the heart are not well supplied by oxygen. Thus the cardiac performance diminishes with prolonged duration of hypertension leading possibly to heart failure. But even in the early stages of hypertension the ventricles become stiffer due to an increased amount of collagen. Their relaxation during diastole, and thus their filling, is impaired. The slower relaxation of the heart muscle prolongs the duration of diastole. The heart rate is therefore lower and as the stroke volume does not change, cardiac output decreases. The number of arterioles in many organs is lower than in subjects with normal pressure and this limits the flow even if the pressure which drives the blood is increased.[23]

The distribution of flow to different organs changes with lower flow to the kidneys, liver, intestines and skin. Although there are fewer arterioles in skeletal muscle of hypertensive rats, flow in individual arterioles is higher than in controls and thus the total blood flow is only slightly lower than in controls. However, the increase during muscle contractions is smaller than in controls. The oxygen and nutrients supply is also lower in spite of the fact that the number of capillaries in skeletal muscles is either not changed or only slightly decreased, and the pressure which forces the flow through them is higher. This may be explained by higher blood flow velocity in individual arterioles and capillaries. The red blood cells thus spend too short a time in capillaries and do not release enough oxygen.

The inadequate increase in blood flow during muscle contraction in hypertension is partly due to the limited capacity of the endothelial cells to produce substances (such as NO) important for dilatation of small (arterioles) as well as larger (brachial) vessels. Another important factor is a higher density of nerve fibres involved in vasoconstriction.

The vasoconstriction as well as the level of noradrenalin (which also causes vasoconstriction), is diminished by moderate endurance training which, consequently, lower blood pressure. Exercise may also reduce the left ventricle hypertrophy and lowers both systolic and diastolic pressures. However, hypertension reappeared after a 1 month rest period even in subjects who had been trained for 9 months. Exercised trained animals had normal muscle blood flow and no deficit in capillary supply. Training also restored exercise-induced increase in blood flow, both in the heart and in skeletal muscle.[24] This was due to elimination of the endothelial dysfunction and to improved generation of NO in small as well as in larger arteries.[13]

Although there are no reports on the long-term effect of electrical stimulation on hypertension, it was shown that only 1 h low frequency stimulation decreased blood pressure in hypertensive rats, possibly due to release of endorphins. It may be that chronic electrical stimulation applied on a longer time basis could be beneficial in the treatment of hypertension.

2.4.3 Heart Failure

Heart failure is an inadequate capacity of the heart to pump enough blood to the periphery to maintain the viability and function of the body organs. It may appear as a result of long-lasting hypertension when the hypertrophy of the cardiac muscle fails to overcome the resistance of the high blood pressure; some of the blood remains in the ventricles expanding them and cardiac output decreases. Another cause of heart failure is leaky heart valves causing some blood that has been expelled from the ventricle to return back to the heart. The volume of the ventricles is then enlarged; this results initially in heart hypertrophy and eventually in heart failure. Heart attack leaves part of the cardiac muscle replaced by scar tissue. Thus the ventricle cannot contract properly and expel the blood to the periphery with consequences described above. Whatever the primary cause, patients with heart failure have lower cardiac output and heart rate, particularly during exercise. In addition, particularly in cases of hypertension, the stiffer aorta does not enlarge to accommodate the blood ejected from the heart with each heart beat.[25] The arteries supplying the limbs in patients with heart failure have also a smaller capacity to dilate and consequently the amount of blood brought to skeletal muscles is smaller than normal, even at rest. The deficit in muscle blood flow is even greater during exercise and this, together with some metabolic and structural changes, such as shift in fibre composition from aerobic to anaerobic muscle fibres causes muscle fatigue on exertion.

The small vessels, arterioles, are narrower, constrict more readily and dilate less. This limits the access of blood to capillaries where the blood flow is more intermittent and slower and thus the supply of the essential substances for maintenance of muscle metabolism is not adequate. In addition, the number of capillaries supplying muscle fibres is decreased. All these factors, taken together, cause, in the long run, the reduction of skeletal muscle mass.[26]

The limited ability of all vessels to dilate is due to the fact that their endothelial lining has a deficient capacity to generate NO.[13] In addition, vessels in skeletal muscles constrict more readily than in normal individuals as the nerve fibres causing contraction of the smooth muscles and thus narrowing of vessels are more active. Indeed, suppression of the high activity of vasoconstrictor fibres in patients with heart failure increased muscle blood flow. In contrast to normal subjects, where blood flow during exercise increases in skeletal muscles and decreases elsewhere, the non-muscle flow remains constant.

Many of the inadequacies of circulation in heart failure can be improved by exercise, particularly by endurance training which has been used for a long time to improve recovery after myocardial infarction. Training decreased the diameter of the enlarged left ventricle, increased stroke volume and diminished the aortic stiffness. It also restored the endothelial dysfunction and thus dilatation of arteries supplying the limbs and the heart, the coronary arteries. Nevertheless, exercising only a small group of muscles had no beneficial effect on endothelial function and thus the capacity of vessels to increase their diameter and blood flow in patients with heart failure, although it was effective in normal subjects.[27]

There are, however, problems with exercise training in heart failure. As the most effective training usually engages a great number of muscles, and thus presents a great demand on the cardiac output, it might not be always possible to use it in people either with advanced heart failure or in elderly patients. As mentioned above, exercise with only a small group of muscles is not very effective. An alternative approach is muscle stimulation. This can be performed in a limited muscle group and for a much longer period of time than voluntary contractions without presenting an increased demand on cardiac output.

Short bursts of high frequency stimulation increased indeed the strength and bulk of thigh muscles in patients with heart failure; low frequency electrical stimulation of thigh and calf muscles increased strength and volume of calf muscles. It also increased blood flow in the femoral artery (supplying the leg muscles), increased oxidative metabolism (which is severely decreased in patients with heart failure) and diminished anaerobic metabolism and improved the walking distance.[28] Stimulation also increases emptying of veins and thus reduces venous pressure. Thus the capillary pressure and the amount of fluid passing out of them is reduced and oedema – a feature of heart failure – is also reduced. Experimental data also demonstrated increased capillary supply in chronically stimulated muscles in rats with heart failure. For some years attempts were made to alleviate the failing force of the cardiac muscle by surgical techniques called cardiomyoplasty when a skeletal muscle was wrapped either around the heart or around the aorta and stimulated at the frequency of the heart beat. However, normal skeletal muscles would rapidly fatigue and would fail to perform sufficiently strong contractions. It was therefore necessary to transform them into slow contracting fatigue resistant muscles. In practice,

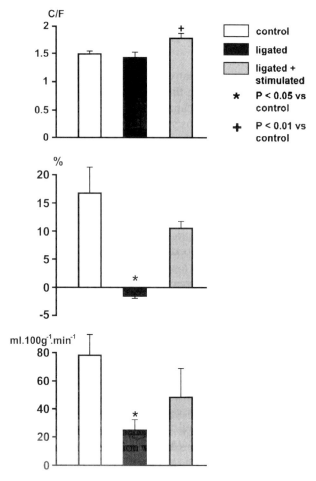

Fig. 2.11 Effect of electrical stimulation on vessels in ischemic muscles. Muscle blood flow to the hind limb was limited by ligation of the main supplying artery to mimic occlusion of the main vessels occurring in patients. Although this procedure did not decrease the capillary supply (top), it eliminated the dilatation of arterioles (middle) and increase in blood flow in contracting muscles. Chronic electrical stimulation (10 impulses per second for 105 min per day, 15 min on, 85 min off) increased capillary supply, restored dilatation of arterioles and increase in muscle blood flow. (From[33] with kind permission of Springer Science and Business Media.)

2.6   Stroke

Stroke (brain damage) occurs when blood flow to a region of the brain is obstructed, or when blood supply is disrupted due to a rupture of an artery in the brain. It is mostly accompanied by increased heart rate, higher blood pressure, lower volume

Chronic stimulation (3xdaily for 20 min) in the in patients with peripheral disease

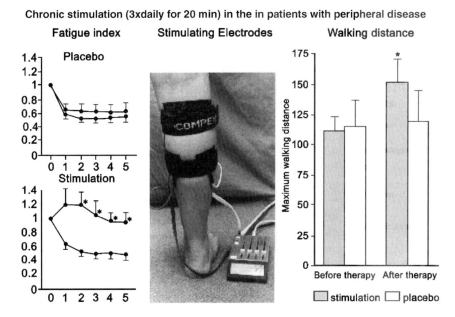

Fig. 2.12 Treatment of patients with peripheral vascular disease by electrical stimulation. Patients stimulated their calf muscles (the position of the electrodes is shown in the middle) three times daily for 20 min (8 impulses per second with palpable contractions but no pain) for 4 weeks. Controls used a stimulator that did not elicit contractions. Maximum walking distance (right) without pain was increased by stimulation but not changed in the control group. Fatigue index (left), measured as a proportion of the force developed by the muscles at the beginning of stimulation at the end of 5 min contractions decreased to 0.4 (60% fatigue) in patients without stimulation and in the control group (black dots), After 4 weeks of stimulation the muscles did not fatigue (red line) and the tension developed at the end of 5 min contractions was similar to that at the beginning. (Based on data from[34] and courtesy of Dr M. D. Brown, School of Sport and Exercise Sciences, University of Birmingham, UK.)

of blood expelled by the heart during each contraction and increased resistance to flow which means that less blood is getting to all organs in the body. Blood flow in skeletal muscles is decreased at rest, and the increase during muscle contractions is smaller. This is to a certain extent due to the impaired endothelial function in large vessels. However, little is known about endothelial function in small vessels and capillaries. Increased level of noradrenalin and increased tone of the vasoconstrictor nerves also play a role in decreasing muscle blood flow.[38]

Both training and electrical stimulation have been used for many years to treat patients suffering from stroke, and both certainly can improve muscle strength, gait and general recovery. However, it is not known to what extent they improve muscle blood flow or capillary supply.

2.7   Oedema

As mentioned previously, oedema is formed when blood cannot leave freely the tissues due to a narrowing or plugging of the veins. It also occurs when capillaries are more leaky to proteins; these accumulate in the tissue outside the vessels and attract water from the vessels. Oedema also takes place when the lymphatic drainage is blocked, as it happens for instance when lymphatic nodes are removed due to cancer. The first situation arises during long standing or sitting without movements, in cases of insufficient venous valves or in heart failure when the right heart cannot pump out the blood which it receives from the periphery. Leaky capillaries occur during inflammation or tissue damage by trauma.

Treatment of oedema must, of course, involve the treatment of the original disease that caused it (as, for instance, in heart failure). Oedema can, however, be always reduced by muscle movements which increase the venous return. Passive movements, active muscle contractions or contractions elicited by electrical stimulation are all helpful. Electrical stimulation of calf muscles could be of great benefit to people on long-haul flights when it is sometimes very difficult to move due to restricted leg space. Electrical stimulation was also used to remove hand oedema in patients with cerebrovascular diseases. It was more effective than limb elevation that reduced the venous pressure only passively.[39]

Electrical stimulation was also applied successfully, but so far only in experiments, in cases of oedema caused by inflammation or histamine which is a substance causing leaky capillaries. The mechanism is not quite clear, but it is possible that it can increase the contractility of the lymphatic vessels and thus accelerate the removal of protein and water from the space outside capillaries.

2.8   Muscle Inactivity and its Consequences

2.8.1   Decreased Muscle Activity

Training or electrical stimulation increase muscle activity and lead to growth of capillaries and an increased size of the vascular bed. It could thus be expected, that decreased activity has the opposite effect. Experimental data show that unloading of antigravitational skeletal muscles (those involved in the maintenance of posture) for 2 weeks caused muscle atrophy with decreased number of capillaries in relation to muscle fibres due to destruction of some endothelial cells. Although there was no change in blood pressure (unlike in hypertension), the arterial wall in vessels outside the affected muscles became thicker and the capability of arteries to dilate was diminished. In contrast, the arteries supplying disused muscles were smaller and blood flow in the affected muscles was lower when the animals returned to their normal standing position. As mentioned several times previously, the friction between moving red blood cells and the endothelial lining of the vessels, the shear stress, is very important in the maintenance of the endothelial function, namely in the activation of a number of processes resulting in the release of NO as well as of other substances important not only in the mediation of vessel widening but also in their growth. Due to lower blood flow the capacity of the endothelial cells to produce NO was decreased and arteries as well as smaller vessels, arterioles, did not dilate in response to various stimuli. Although not yet explored, similar changes may occur during space fights. It would be impossible to prevent these changes by training, but electrical stimulation may prevent them – a field that has to be explored.[40]

Another type of immobilisation, linked with injuries, such as plaster casts or metal pins also result in muscle wasting but not necessarily in loss of capillaries. As muscle fibres become smaller, the distance between capillaries diminishes, and, if immobilization does not last for a very long time, the actual proportion of capillaries supplying individual muscle fibres decreases relatively little. However, a small proportion of capillaries have damaged endothelium. Blood flow in immobilized muscles is lower and increases less when the demand for oxygen is increased. Experimental work showed that electrical stimulation prevented muscle atrophy and loss of capillaries in muscles immobilized by casts. However, its effect on the changes in muscle circulation is still not quite clear.[41]

2.8.2   Denervation (Disruption of the Nerves)

Whenever the nerves supplying muscles are interrupted or damaged, muscles can no longer be activated and undergo atrophy. However, blood flow during the first 1–2 months after denervation is similar to control muscles because the size of the vascular bed remains relatively constant while the bulk of the muscle fibres diminishes. Velocity of flow in capillaries is actually increased, possibly because the arterioles are dilated due to release of dilating metabolites from the degenerating muscle fibres. Loss of capillaries after long-lasting denervation[42] is linked to a decreased level of various growth factors. Changes in arterioles appear with prolonged time after denervation particularly in glycolytic parts of muscles. Electrical stimulation has been used to alleviate muscle atrophy after denervation but its possible role on capillary growth after nerve disruption has still to be explored.

2.8.3   Diseases of Muscle

Although there are many forms of muscle diseases, relatively little is known about the changes in blood vessels.

Duchenne dystrophy (named after the person who described it in the second half of the 19th century), is a hereditary disease characterised by gradual muscle wasting including muscles involved in respiration leading to death in the second or third decade of life. Muscle blood flow or capillary supply does not seem to be impaired, but alterations in the capillary ultrastructure (e.g. endothelial cell swelling, narrower lumen) have been described. These could contribute to a limited capillary transport capacity.[43] Other muscle diseases due to inflammation have lower capillary supply. However, there is no data on the effect of electrical stimulation on microcirculation in any of these diseases.

2.8.4 *Spinal Cord Injuries*

The changes in the function of the heart and blood pressure are different in individual patients and vary with the site of injury. Experimental data showed that alterations of the heart rate and blood pressure were different in injuries occurring in the upper or lower part of the spinal cord. Patients with damage at the level of upper thoracic vertebrae resulting in paralysis of upper as well as lower limbs (tetraplegia) had decreased heart rate and blood pressure. However, with damage at a lower level which leads to paralysis of only the lower part of the body (paraplegia), heart rate and blood pressure increased. The higher the level of injury, the lower the blood pressure. Patients with tetraplegia had relatively small heart ventricles, smaller cardiac output and lower systolic, diastolic and mean pressure. Cardiac output is lower in tetraplegic as well as in paraplegic patients with lesions in the lower thoracic region of the spinal cord, both at rest and during electrically induced muscle contractions. On passive standing (assisted by an electrically operated system) cardiac output, stroke volume and blood pressure decreased even more. Electrical stimulation of the calf muscles during standing activated the venous pump in contracting muscles and thus increased venous return and prevented the reduction of cardiac output. It also helped to normalise the blood pressure.[44]

Blood flow in thigh muscles was lower in patients with damage at higher levels due to a higher tone of sympathetic vasoconstrictor fibres. The diameter of the femoral artery was smaller and consequently increase in blood flow, either after temporary arrest of blood supply (reactive hyperaemia) or in response to muscle contractions elicited by electrical stimulation was also smaller than in normal subjects. Changes in the diameter of arteries and in muscle blood flow appeared within 3 weeks after the injury and remained constant during the following months. Most of these differences could be eliminated by electrical stimulation of thigh muscle. Stimulation increased the muscle fibre oxidative capacity and normalized the decreased capillary supply.[45] (Fig. 2.13).The vascular bed in the body above the level of injury was not affected: the diameters of the brachial and carotid arteries did not change.

Although there is no data on blood flow in stimulated paralyzed muscles, it is possibly higher at least during muscle contractions. That would mean that the capacity of the endothelium of the vessel to generate NO and thus preserve normal endothelial function would be improved with stimulation. This seems indeed to be the case. Normal endothelial function is essential in preventing thrombus formation.

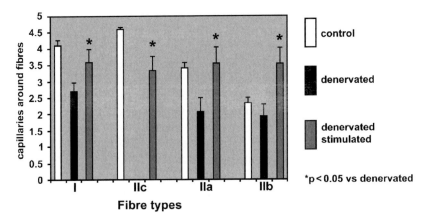

Fig. 2.13 Number of capillaries around muscle fibres. The number of capillaries around muscle fibres of different fibre types in a thigh muscle of normal people, in muscles of patients with muscle atrophy after spinal cord lesion denervated and in patients with spinal cord lesion whose muscle were electrically stimulated for 10 weeks. (Values for control muscles based on data from[46] and values for denervated and denervated stimulated from[43].)

Thrombosis is more frequent in patients with spinal cord injury and was prevented by short lasting (60 min) electrical stimulation of calf muscles.[47]

2.9 Wound Healing

Electrical stimulation has been used only in the treatment of wounds of the skin. Therefore the process of wound healing is described only in this tissue.

The simplest form of wound is surgical wound after an operation. Healing is dependent on growth of new vessels which is preceded by a sequence of events. Disruption of vessels, be it in surgical wound, in an ulcer or in bed sores, leads to some bleeding, coagulation of blood and filling of the wound with fibrin – a substance formed in blood clots. White blood cells start to migrate to the fibrin clot to remove the debris very soon afterwards. After only a few days they are replaced by another type of white blood cells which contain growth factors that stimulate growth of new capillaries. At the same time, cells at the edge of the wound called fibroblasts start to divide and produce collagen, a protein which strengthens the wound edges and forms the scar tissue. Capillaries in surgical wounds appear about 2 days after surgery and are gradually transformed into large vessels so that the vascularization is completed within 6–7 days. Capillary growth is faster when the levels of oxygen are increased by exposing the wound to high oxygen pressures while wound healing is impaired in situations with low blood flow, such as in patients with extensive bleeding, low blood pressure or ischemia. On the other hand, increased blood flow, whether by heat, by compression and decompression (which increase the venous pump) or by growth factors or factors that produce dilatation, improves wound healing.

Electrical stimulation has been used as a method to accelerate wound healing although the mechanism is still not understood. It has been demonstrated that there is a negative electrical potential in the wound during the phase of healing and that direct current with the negative electrode close to the wound accelerates migration and proliferation of fibroblasts and collagen synthesis and thus increases the strength of the connective tissue forming the scar. Capillary blood flow was improved and the size of the wound rapidly decreased with direct current stimulation. The increase in flow is probably due to vasodilating peptides (calcitonin gene related peptide or substance P) which might be released from the stimulation of sensory nerves. Stimulation decreased oedema and accelerated removal of the debris from wounds, a process which is particularly important in healing of bed sores or ulcers. Different other types of stimulation (asymmetric biphasic pulses, low frequency sinusoidal current) and low or high frequency were also used. It can be concluded that various forms of electrical stimulation have been shown to accelerate healing of different kinds of wounds, and there is a general consent that electrical stimulation increases flow and stimulates proliferation of various categories of cells involved in wound healing. However the exact mechanism is still not known. In cases of venous ulcers, electrical stimulation may be successful as it increases the function of the venous pump.[48]

2.10   Conclusions: Comparison Between the Effects of Training and Electrical Stimulation in Disease

The main cardiovascular effects of endurance training occur in skeletal muscles and in the heart with increased capillary supply and the whole vascular bed in both tissues. Blood flow increases only in skeletal muscle and only during maximal performance. The heart hypertrophies, stroke volume increases and heart rate is lower. In contrast, stimulation does not appreciably alter the cardiac function, but has a greater effect on skeletal muscles with a much faster and greater increase in capillary supply and increased blood flow even at rest. Both training end electrical stimulation increase the ability of vessels to dilate due to increased generation of NO and other factors by the endothelial cells. The effect is restricted to the stimulated muscles while training improves endothelial function in most vessels including the aorta.

Endurance training improves endothelial function also in old age. It improves capillary supply in oxidative skeletal muscles and reduces the stiffness of the aorta. Stimulation increases capillary supply only in the treated muscles, but as it preferentially induces capillary growth in fast glycolytic muscles (where it is impaired during aging and is the cause of fatigue), it has a potential use in old people. Both procedures improve endothelial function.

The beneficial effect of training in hypertension has been long recognised. It can diminish heart hypertrophy and lower both systolic and diastolic pressure. It restores the deficit in arteriolar and capillary numbers and the capacity to increase muscle blood flow during contractions. The latter is to a great extent due to the correction of the endothelial dysfunction in most vessels resulting from hypertension. The effect of long-term electrical stimulation in hypertension has so far not been reported.

Training has been used successfully for a long time to enhance the function of the heart after myocardial infarction. It is also used in other types of heart failure where the physical fatigue is partly due to the inadequate supply of blood to skeletal muscles. The beneficial effect is mainly due to the correction of the endothelial dysfunction in all vessels and therefore improved vasodilatation. It can also increase stroke volume. However, these effects occur only when the training includes large groups of muscle and this, of course, increases the demand on the heart function. Thus the effect of training is beneficial only in a mild form of heart failure. In contrast, electrical stimulation increases muscle strength and blood flow, improves venous return and can reduce limb oedema without increasing the demand on the heart.

Training is acknowledged as the most effective type of therapy in PVD. However, as these diseases are usually connected with arteriosclerosis and possible problems with diminished heart performance, it is important to find therapy which would not increase demand on the heart (and training certainly does that). Electrical stimulation is definitively a therapy of choice. It can be used in one leg only thus improving walking distance. It improves muscle blood flow, corrects the endothelial dysfunction and thus the capacity of vessels to dilate and it diminishes muscle fatigue.

Similarly, electrical stimulation can be used in the treatment of oedema whether in heart failure (see above), in stroke patients or during long-haul flights. It is also used as a therapy for various types of immobilisation (casts, denervation, decreased muscle activity due to lack of gravitational forces, spinal cord injuries) where the use of endurance training is not applicable and where it can improve the endothelial dysfunction.

Acknowledgement I would like to thank my collaborators, particularly to Dr. M.D. Brown, through all the years and to Dr. Gillian E. Knight, for all her help.

References

1. B. Folkow, and E. Neil, *Circulation* (Oxford University Press, Oxford, 1971).
2. J. A. G. Rhodin, *Handbook of Physiology, Cardiovascular System, Vol II* (American Physiological Society, Bethesda, 1980).
3. O. Hudlicka, M. D. Brown, and S. Egginton, The microcirculation in skeletal muscle in: *Myology, Basic and Clinical, 3rd edition*, edited by A. G. Engel and C. Franzini-Armstrong (McGraw-Hill, New York, 2004), pp. 511–533.
4. J. R. Levick, *An Introduction to Cardiovascular Physiology* (Arnold Publishers, London, 2003).

5. K. K. Kallioski, C. Scheede-Bergdahl, M. Kjaer, and R. Boushel, Muscle perfusion and metabolic heterogeneity: insights from noninvasive imaging techniques, *Exerc. Sport Sci. Rev.* **34**:164–170 (2006).

6. R. Myrhage, and O. Hudlicka, The microvascular bed and capillary surface area in rat extensor hallucis proprius muscle (EHP), *Microvasc. Res.* **11**:315–323 (1976).

7. M. H. Laughlin, Cardiovascular responses to exercise, *Am. J. Physiol.* **277**:S244–259 (1999).

8. S. S. Segal, and S. E. Bearden, Organisation and control of circulation to skeletal muscle, in: *ACSM's Advanced Exercise Physiology*, edited by C. T. Tipton (Lippincot, Williams & Wilkins, Philadelphia, 2006), pp. 343–356.

9. M. H. Laughlin, Distribution of skeletal muscle blood flow during locomotory exercise, *Adv. Exp. Med. Biol.* **227**:87–101 (1988).

10. C. G. Blomqvist, and B. Saltin, Cardiovascular adaptations to physical training, *Annu. Rev. Physiol.* **45**:169–189 (1983).

11. O. Hudlicka, and M. D. Brown, Modulators of angiogenesis, in: *Angiogenesis in Health and Disease*, edited by G. M. Rubanyi (Marcel Decker, New York, 2000), pp. 215–244.

12. O. Hudlicka, M. D. Brown, and S. Egginton, Angiogenesis in skeletal and cardiac muscle, *Physiol. Rev.* **72**:369–417 (1992).

13. N. M. Moyna, and P. D. Thompson, The effect of physical activity on endothelial function in man, *Acta Physiol. Scand.* **180**:113–123 (2004).

14. O. Hudlicka, M. D. Brown, S. May, A. Zakrzewicz, and A. R. Pries, Changes in capillary shear stress in skeletal muscles exposed to long- term activity: role of NO, *Microcirculation* **13**:249–59 (2006).

15. M. D. Brown, M. A. Cotter, O. Hudlicka, and G. Vrbova, The effects of different patterns of muscle activity on capillary density, mechanical properties and structure of slow and fast rabbit muscles. *Pflugers Arch. Eur. J. Physiol.* **361**:241–50 (1976).

16. J. M. Dawson, and O. Hudlicka, The effect of long-term activity on the microvasculature of rat glycolytic skeletal muscle, *Int. J. Microcirc. Clin. Exper.* **8**:53–69 (1989).

17. M. D. Brown, S. Jeal, J. Bryant, and J. Gamble, Modification of microvasculaar filtration capacity in human limbs by training and electrical stimulation, *Acta Physiol. Scand.* **173**:359–368 (2001).

18. P. D. Fagri, J. J. Votto, and C. F. Hovorka, Venous dynamics in the lower extremities in response to electrical stimulation, *Arch. Phys. Med. Rehabil.* **79**:842–848 (1998).

19. I. O. Man, G. S. Lepar, M. C. Morrisey, and J. K. Cywinski, Effect of neuromussclular electrical stimulation on foot/ankle volume during standing, *Med. Sci. Sport. Exerc.* **35**:630–634 (2003).

20. M. Cabric, H. J. Appell, and A. Resic, Stereological analysis of capillaries in electrostimulated human muscles. *Int. J. Sports. Med.* **8**:327–330 (1987).

21. A. U. Ferrari, A. Radaelli, and M. Centola, Invited review: aging and the role of the cardiovascular system. *J. Appl. Physiol.* **95**:2591–7 (2003).

22. B. A. Harris, The influence of endurance and resistance exercise in muscle capillarisation in the elderly: a review. *Acta Physiol. Scand.* **185**:89–97 (2005).

23. B. Folkow, Pathophysiology of hypertension. *J. Hypertension* **11**:S21–S24 (1993).

24. J. M. Hagberg, J. J. Park, and M. D. Brown, The role of exercise training in the treatment of hypertension: an update, *Sports. Med.* **30**:193–206 (2000).

25. P. Rerkpattanpipat, W. G. Hudndley, K. M. Link, P. H. Brubaker, C. A. Hamilton, S. N. Darty, T. M. Morgan, and D. W. Kitzman, Relation of aortic distensibility determined by magnetic resonance imaging in patients > or = 60 years of age to systolic heart failure and exercise capacity to systolic heart failure and exercise capacity, *Am. J. Cardiol.* **90**:1221–1225 (2002).

26. B. D. Duscha, F. W. Kraus, S. J. Ketevian, M. J. Sullivan, H. J. Green, F. H. Schachat, A. M. Pippen, C. A. Brawner, J. M. Blank, and B. H. Annex, Capillary density of skeletal muscle: a contributing mechanism for exercise intolerance in class II-III chronic heart failure independent of other peripheral alterations, *J. Am. Coll. Cardiol.* **33**:1956–1963 (1999).

27. M. D. Witham, A. D. Struthers, and M. E. McMurdo, Exercise training as a therapy for chronic heart failure: can older people benefit? *J. Am. Geriatr. Soc.* **51**:699–709 (2003).

28. J. F. Maillefert, J. C. Eicher, P. Walker, I. Rouhier-Marcer, F. Branley, M. Cohen, F. Brunotte, J. E. Wolf, J. M. Casillas, and J. P. Didier, Effects of low-frequency electrical stimulation on quadricepss and calf muscles in patients with chronic heart failure, *J. Cardiopulm. Rehabil.* **18**:277–282 (1998).

29. C. J. Kelsall, M. D. Brown, J. Kent, M. Kloehn, and O. Hudlicka, Arteriolar endothelial dysfunction is restored in ischaemic muscles by chronic electrical stimulation, *J. Vasc. Res.* **41**:241–251 (2004).

30. N. C. Hickey, O. Hudlicka, P. Gosling, C. P. Shearman, and M. H. Simms, Intermittent claudication incites systemic neutrophil activation and increased vascular permeability, *Br. J. Surg.* **80**:181–184 (1993).

31. P. V. Tisi, and C. P. Shearman, The evidence for exercise-induced inflammation in intermittent claudication. Should we encourage patients to walk? *Eur. J. Vasc. Endovasc. Surg.* **15**:7–17 (1998).

32. O. Hudlicka, M. D. Brown, S. Egginton, and J. M. Dawson, Effect of long-term electrical stimulation on vascular supply and fatigue in chronically ischemic muscles, *J. Appl. Physiol.* **77**:1317–1324 (1994).

33. O. Hudlicka, and M. D. Brown, Hemodynamic forces, exercise and angiogenesis, in: *Therapeutic Angiogenesis*, edited by J. A. Dormandy, W. P. Dole and G. M. Rubanyi (Springer-Verlag, Berlin, Heidelberg, 1999), pp. 87–123.

34. G. M. Tsang, M. A. Green, A. J. Crow, F. C. Smith, S. Beck, O. Hudlicka, and C. P. Shearman, Chronic muscle stimulation improves ischaemic muscle performance in patients with peripheral vascular disease, *Eur. J. Vasc. Surg.* **8**:419–427 (1994).

35. S. I. Anderson, P. Whatling, O. Hudlicka, P. Gosling, M. Simms, and M. D. Brown, Chronic transcutaneous electrical stimulation of calf muscles improves functional capacity without inducing systemic inflammation in claudicants, Eur J Vasc Endovasc Surg. **27**:201–209 (2004).

36. M. A. Oldfield, M. Simms, and M. D. Brown, Microvascular filtration capacity is modified by chronic stimulation in ischemic human limbs without changes in local vascular control, *Microcirculation* **12**:666 (2005).

37. A. J. Clover, M. J. McCarthy, K. Hodgkinson, P. R. Bell, and N. P. Brindle, Noninvasive augmentation of microvessel number in patients with peripheral vascular disease, *J. Vasc. Surg.* **38**:1309–1312 (2003).

38. M. F. McCarthy, Up-regulation of endothelial nitric oxide activity as a central strategy for prevention of ischemic stroke – just say No to stroke! *Med. Hypothesis* **55**:386–403 (2000).

39. P. D. Faghri, The effects of neuromuscular stimulation-induced muscle contractions versus elevation on hand edema in CVA patients, *J. Hand. Ther.* **10**:29–34 (1997).

40. M. D. Delp, M. Brown, M. H. Laughlin, and E. M. Hasser, Rat aortic vasoreactivity is altered by old age and limb unloading, *J. Appl. Physiol.* **78**:2079–2086 (1995).

41. D. A. Lake, Neuromuscular electrical stimulation. An overview and it's application in the treatment of sports injuries, *Sports Med.* **13**:320–336 (1992).

42. A. B. Borisov, S. K. Huang, and B. M. Carlson, Remodelling of the vascular bed and progressive loss of capillaries in denervated skeletal muscle, *Anat. Record* **258**:292–304 (2000).

43. R. M. Crameri, A. Weston, M. Climstein, G. M. Davis, and J. R. Sutton, Effects of electrical stimulation-induced leg training on skeletal muscle adaptability in spinal cord injury, *Scand. J. Med. Sci. Sports* **12**:316–322 (2002).

44. H. Leinonen, J. Juntunen, H. Somer, and J. Rapola, Capillary circulation and morphology in Duchenne muscular dystrophy, *Eur. Neurol.* **18**:249–255 (1979).

45. F. Dela, T. Mohr, C. M. Jensen, H. L. Haahr, N. H. Sechenr, F. Biering-Sorensen, and M. Kjaer, Cardiovascular control during exercise: insights from spinal cord-injured humans, *Circulation* **107**:2127–2133 (2003).

46. F. Ingjer, Effects of endurance training on muscle fibre ATP-ase activity, capillary supply and mitochondrial content in man, *J. Physiol (London)* **294**:419–432 (1979).

47. J. L. Olive, J. M. Slade, J. A. Dudley, and K. K. McCully, Blood flow and muscle fatigue in SCI individuals during electrical stimulation, *J. Appl. Physiol.* **94**:701–708 (2003).

48. K. M. Bogie, S. I. Reger, S. P. Levine, and V. Saghal, Electrical stimulation for pressure sore prevention and wound healing, *Assist. Technol.* **12**:50–66 (2000).

Chapter 3
Electrical Stimulation as a Therapeutic Tool to Restore Motor Function

Gerta Vrbová[1], Olga Hudlicka[2], and Kristin Schaefer Centofanti[3]

Abstract Electrical stimulation of muscles and nerves to improve recovery of function is used in the following conditions: (1) after injury to the joints or muscles. It appears that in these cases electrical stimulation can restore motor functions more quickly and more completely then in the absence of this intervention or following voluntary exercise. (2) Following damage to the central or peripheral nervous system or during muscle diseases; motor functions can be improved by electrical stimulation of muscles or nerves. Electrical stimulation has been most widely used after spinal cord injury. Moreover, particularly designed methods of stimulation of muscles of spinal cord injury patients are able to initiate and control the lost movements. In patients with stroke and head injuries electrical stimulation can also help to restore function. (3) The consequences of inactivity as a result of long lasting bed rest are also successfully counteracted by electrical stimulation of muscles. Moreover, lack of gravity, such as during space flight, leads to changes of the neuromuscular system that resemble those during bed rest, and these too can be successfully treated by electrical stimulation.

Keywords Electrical stimulation, knee injuries, neurological disorders, muscle diseases, bed rest, space flight

3.1 Introduction

The previous two chapters summarise results to show that muscle properties as well as their blood flow can be modified by electrical stimulation applied by external devices. In view of these findings it is clear that this approach may be beneficial

[1] Autonomic Neuroscience Centre, Royal Free and University College Medical School, Rowland Hill Street, London NW3 2PF

[2] Department of Physiology, University of Birmingham Medical School, Birmingham B15 TT UK

[3] JKC Research Partnership, London E5 8AP, UK

G. Vrbová et al., *Application of Muscle/Nerve Stimulation in Health and Disease*,
© Springer Science + Business Media B.V. 2008

both for improving the function of normal human muscles and for maintaining and restoring movement in different conditions where due to various insults the normal function of muscles is prevented or altered.

It is well known that inactivity (disuse) of skeletal muscles leads to their wasting, increased fatigability, and often irreversible structural damage. In people who leave a sedentary life, electrical stimulation of their muscles (EMS), or stimulation of muscles via their nerves (NMES) can restore muscle tone, strength and fatigue resistance in a similar way as voluntary exercise program. Indeed, recent research indicates that both methods of stimulation can bring about improvements of muscle function and structure faster and more efficiently than conventional exercise (see Chapter 4).

In this chapter we will discuss the use of electrical stimulation for restoring muscle function and structural integrity in conditions leading to prolonged forced inactivity such as (1) injury to joints and muscles as a result of accidents or sport activities, (2) disease or damage to the central or peripheral nervous system or the muscles themselves so that the person is unable to carry out voluntary movement, (3) inactivity as a consequence of systemic diseases when the patient is bedridden or unable to move. We will summarize the evidence that shows that in all three conditions electrical stimulation can replace the missing natural activity.

3.2 Muscle Stimulation to Aid Recovery After Injuries to Joints and Muscles

Following injuries to joints and muscles the injured parts of the body are often immobilized for some time to allow the damaged joints and muscles to heal. While immobilisation is usually necessary, it has deleterious consequences on the function of muscles, and recovery is often slow because muscles have deteriorated during the period of immobilisation. It is in these cases that electrical stimulation of muscles during the period of immobilisation and afterwards is beneficial and speeds up recovery.

The most thoroughly explored condition is that after knee injury, particularly after the rupture of the anterior cruciate ligament. This injury affects young active people, and is usually a result of exercise. Traditionally, the leg is immobilized and often surgery has to be carried out to re-suture the anterior cruciate ligament. Interestingly, even months after surgery the thigh muscles, particularly the quadriceps muscles, do not regain their normal strength, which for active individuals is a disadvantage.[1] There is much evidence that when the quadriceps muscles are electrically stimulated during the period of immobilisation and subsequent recuperation, the recovery of force of the muscle is more complete and the period of restricted movement shorter than without this intervention[2] (see Table 3.1).

In most cases of knee immobilisation NMES is effective in preventing the decrease in muscle strength, muscle mass and the oxidative capacity of thigh muscles. Most studies indicate that it is more effective in preventing muscle atrophy when compared to no exercise, isometric exercise of the quadriceps muscle group, isometric co-contractions of both hamstrings and quadriceps groups and combined isometric exercise.[3] In these studies electrical stimulation was carried out using percutaneous stimulation and no invasive methods were necessary. Knee injuries affect 80% of sports people, particularly those engaged in rugby or football and it follows that even in cases where surgery is not necessary, a period of enforced rest will quickly lead to muscle deterioration. A programme of rehabilitation using NMES to strengthen the quadriceps can vastly accelerate the rate of recovery of the leg and its use.[4] Table 1 summarises results obtained by various types of stimulation on recovering of function after knee injury.

Inactivity of other joints of both upper and lower limbs are likely to have similar effects on the muscles involved in movement of these joints as that described for quadriceps, i.e. they become atrophic, produce less force and are fatigable. Their recovery is likely to be more complete and faster if electrical stimulation is used both during and after immobilisation.

When specific parts of the body need to be immobilised for long periods of time in a cast or brace due to a fracture of bone, tears of ligaments or tendons, in order to allow healing of the damaged area to take place, stimulation of the muscles by placing self adhesive electrodes under the cast or brace or into the opening of the cast will prevent development of the detrimental changes and help to follow a more intensive rehabilitation regime later on.

Unfortunately, these approaches and avenues of treatment are not sufficiently explored and not used frequently enough in spite of the fact that recent knowledge about the ability of muscle to respond to electrical stimulation and its beneficial effects on muscle properties have been so clearly documented (see Chapters 1 and 2).

3.3   Muscle Stimulation During Disease or Injury to the CNS and/or Muscle

3.3.1   Neurological Disorders

There is evidence to show that in some neurological conditions such as multiple sclerosis, stroke and particularly spinal cord injury skeletal muscles atrophy and become very fatigable. Electrical stimulation of such affected muscles can either prevent or reverse these changes.[5,6] The benefit of the maintenance of the muscles in good condition may not be immediately obvious since in many neurological disorders the problem is the inability of the person concerned to use the muscle, and the muscle atrophy and fatigability is the result of this lack of use. Nevertheless there are distinct benefits to maintaining the muscles in good condition. These vary with the specific disability the person is suffering from. To give but a few examples:

for patients with multiple sclerosis the better condition of their muscles may mean that they could use them more readily during remission and this would allow the patients to return sooner to normal activities.

Indeed, there is some evidence that in patients with multiple sclerosis following NMES the lower limbs showed an increase in range of movement, and the majority of patients could walk faster following NMES.[7]

3.3.2 *Spinal Cord Injury*

Following spinal cord injury the muscles below the injury are not used, or used inappropriately. This is due to the fact that the connections between the parts of the brain that initiate and control the movement and the neurones that are responsible for giving the command to the muscles to execute the movement are disrupted. According to the type of the injury different symptoms and disturbances of movement develop but in most cases muscle deterioration and fatigability occur.[5] It is important to assess the patients' clinical condition to devise the correct use of electrical stimulation and choice of muscles that need stimulation. Once established which muscles are affected by the spinal cord injury, their deterioration can be prevented or their function restored by well chosen regimens of electrical stimulation.

It is important for the muscles paralysed after spinal cord injury to be kept in good condition, for later on the patients may be trained to carry out movements using various programs of rehabilitation. For these functions the muscles used in the movement need to be able to develop reasonable forces and be resistant to fatigue. Table 1 summarises the effects of different patterns of stimulation used in rehabilitation of patients with spinal cord injury.

The treatment known as functional electrical stimulation (FES) uses either the muscles themselves or the remaining neural circuitry of the damaged spinal cord to achieve movement, in the case of lower limbs standing and walking. When the muscles themselves are stimulated movement is achieved by sequential stimulation of various muscle groups in a pattern that resembles normal movement. In preparation for this training electrical stimulation of the muscles that enables them to gain sufficient strength and fatigue resistance is necessary before the start of the FES training. Once established the FES itself maintains the muscles condition.

Restoration of movement of patients with spinal cord injury by FES was attempted in the 70's by Vodovnik and colleagues.[8] The first trials to elicit a specific movement by muscle stimulation was dorsiflexion of the ankle joint (lifting the toes off the floor) during the swing phase when the leg is off the ground and moving forward during the walking cycle so as to prevent the foot from being dragged. This was achieved by stimulating the muscles of the front of the calf by special devices that regulated the onset of the stimulation by a switch on the heel of the patient which turns on the stimulator during walking just before the beginning of the swing phase of the movement. There is a vast literature on the subject, and the use of different devices using percutaneous stimulation as well as various complicated implantable devices, and feedback loops. A recent review summarizes the available technology.[6]

Functional electrical stimulation has also been used successfully for combined control of elbow extension and hand grasp in C5 and C6 tetraplegics.[9]

In most patients where electrical stimulation of muscles has been used the muscles in question are innervated and although they can not be activated voluntarily by the person in question they can be activated by stimulating their motor nerve

Table 3.1 Examples of parameters of electrical stimulation used in the treatment of spinal cord injuries and immobilisation

Spinal cord injury			
Lesion	Details of stimulation	Effect	Reference
C_6-Th_{12}	Glutei, vastus, hamstrings 30 Hz, 5 s on, 10 s off	Improved strength	39
	16 Hz, 2 s on, 10 s off	Improved endurance	
	15–30 min/day in week 1 up to 120 min/day in week 8	Improved transcutaneous pO_2	
C_6-Th_4	Low frequency (10 Hz), 5 s on, 5 s off	Increased endurance	40
C_6-Th_4	As above	Enhanced oxidative capacity, increased % of type I fibres and C/F	41
	35 Hz, 30 min/day 10 weeks	Increased capillaries around fibres, increased % type I fibres	42
Paraplegia	35 Hz, 11 s on, 60 s off, 30 min	Assisted standing	43
Tetraplegia	No details	Prevention of decrease of blood pressure on passive standing	
	30 Hz, 11 s on, 60 s off, 60 min	Increased venous return decreased blood clotting	44
	50 mA increasing to 150 mA for 30 min 2–3/week for 4 weeks	Increased leg blood flow and femoral artery diameter	45
Immobilisation			
Knee surgery	40 Hz, 0.3 msec biphasic rectangular	Smaller reduction in muscle fibre area	46
Knee surgery	30 Hz, 2 s on, 10 s off, 1 h/day 6 weeks	Smaller loss of muscle bulk	47
Knee surgery	High intensity stimulation	70% increased strength	3
	Low intensity stimulation	51% increased strength	
	Exercise	57% increased strength of quadriceps	
Bed rest			
30 days	60 Hz, for 4 s, 4 × 5 min, with 10 min intervals, 3 days on, 1 day off	Attenuated decrease in fibre cross sectional area and strength, smaller decrease in oxidative capacity	48

either percutaneously or by implanted electrodes. Movement is therefore elicited through the normal nerve-muscle connection, and the muscle is made to contract in response to its neural input (see Chapter 1). Even if paralysed such innervated muscles maintain their ability to respond to electrical stimulation of their motor nerves. This is a great advantage, for the excitability (i.e. response to an electrical stimulus) of nerves is much lower, i.e. less current is needed, than that of muscles. It is much more difficult to achieve contractions of muscles that have lost their nerves and are denervated. Electrical pulses of much higher intensity have to be used to produce contractions of denervated muscles, and this often causes pain and discomfort to the patient.

3.3.3   Denervated Muscles

Nevertheless, in a group of spinal cord injury patients that damaged their motor nerves, and because of the nature of the injury also lost their perception of pain below the lesion, it was found that by using a very special method of electrical stimulation, muscle strength and bulk can be restored even in long term denervated human muscles.[10] In order to elicit contractions of denervated muscles, pulses of longer duration and higher amplitude that provide more current need to be used. Moreover, electrical pulses that take a long time to reach peak amplitude are more effective, unlike for stimulation of innervated muscle where pulses that reach peak amplitude rapidly are favoured. As concluded in a study by Kern et al.[11] "our results show that denervated muscle in humans is indeed trainable and can perform functional activities with FES. Furthermore this method of stimulation can assist in decubitus prevention and significantly improve the mobility of paraplegics". Consistent with these results is the work of Mödlin et al.[12] on stimulation of denervated muscles which reports marked increase of muscle mass and improvement of the condition of muscles in the denervated lower limbs.

3.3.4   Stroke and Head Injuries

After stroke, when parts of the body are paralysed, skeletal muscles deteriorate rapidly. In this situation too, electrical stimulation of the paralysed muscles can help to keep them in a condition where they can be used and help the patient to move.

Since, in stroke patients and after head injury, the upper limb is also affected, electrical stimulation of muscles of the upper limb is recommended.[13] A particular complication of stroke patients is damage to the shoulder joint, i.e. partial dislocation. Electrical stimulation of the muscles of the shoulder girdle can correct the displacement and allow the recovery of movement of the shoulder joint.[14] Stroke is the number one cause of disability in the USA, and positive effects of stimulation are not only encouraging but very important. Newsam and Baker[15] showed that electrical stimulation facilitation programme significantly improved motor unit recruitment in muscles of patients after cerebrovascular accidents. In so far as the mechanisms of improvement are concerned, it has been suggested that the sensory nerves are also excited during the stimulation and this excitation may elicit central nervous system responses important for voluntary recruitment of motor pathways.[16]

3.3.5   Electrical Stimulation to Achieve Artificial Respiration and Control of the Urinary Bladder

In some spinal cord and head injury patients the lesion affects the function of the respiratory muscles, in particular the diaphragm. In these persons it is possible to achieve artificial respiratory support by stimulating the diaphragm via its phrenic nerve. In this case the electrodes have to be implanted so as to get access to the phrenic nerve and this is an invasive procedure. This method of artificial ventilation has been very successful.[17] There are now several phrenic nerve pacing systems commercially available.

Another condition where special devices for electrical stimulation are being used is urinary bladder function.[18] Disturbances of bladder function are quite common after spinal cord injury and again using various implantable devices a better bladder function can be achieved by electrical stimulation. However, their use should be preceded by non implanted devices.[19]

3.3.6   Neuromuscular Diseases

Finally, in some neuromuscular diseases where the muscles themselves are affected and movement is impossible due to their malfunction, as in the case of children with Duchenne and Becker muscular dystrophy, electrical stimulation can be applied to improve the function of diseased muscles. Studies of boys with Duchenne muscular dystrophy show that the progressive deterioration of their muscles, typical of this condition, was halted when their muscles were electrically stimulated using low frequency stimulation.[20] However, only slow frequency electrical stimulation was effective; using higher frequencies of stimulation had no effect.[21] Some of these results were confirmed in studies by Zupan and colleagues,[22,23] where boys who had their muscles stimulated in one leg for 9 months showed a slower rate of deterioration of force of the stimulated muscles than that of the unstimulated muscles in the other leg.

As explained in Chapter 1 (plasticity of the motor unit) of this book, activity can modify gene expression of skeletal muscle fibres, and the pattern of activity delivered

Sometimes research follows indirect routes: although there are millions of patients that at any one time are bed ridden because of illness or accidents, and the deteriorating effect this enforced inactivity has on muscles has been known for a long time, most of the research into using electrical stimulation for helping muscular recovery and reversing the loss of muscle bulk has been carried out on astronauts. There are many similarities between the effect of space flight and bed rest on the human body, and some exciting results on the beneficial effects electrical stimulation during space flight and bed rest have been reported.

Russian researchers used electrical stimulation during simulated weightlessness. Subjects on enforced bed rest received stimulation on their abdominal region, back, thigh and shin, twice a day for 25–30 min. After 45 days, "morphological studies showed a positive effect of electrostimulation on the muscle tissue, preventing the development of atrophic changes".[31] Cherepakin et al.[32] concluded that electrostimulation of muscles increased their strength and tolerance to static loads and prevented their atrophy although a combination of electrical muscle stimulation and physical exercise was necessary to maintain the cardiovascular system.

In 1996, the crew of Columbia space shuttle carried out some experiments on the human musculoskeletal system monitoring muscle activity and used a special device for muscle stimulation. A year later, in 1997, the software of a FES (Functional Electrical Stimulation) device used to elicit movement of muscles in spinal cord injury patients, was merged with the control system of a robot used by astronauts in space, termed by NASA the Remote Manipulator System (NASA, STI, Spinoffs).

In a pilot experiment on astronauts on the Russian MIR space station, a stimulation device via electrodes fitted to specially designed trousers that enabled simultaneous stimulation of 4 muscle groups for 6 h a day was designed and tested. It was concluded that "the synchronous activation of antagonists of the thigh and lower leg prevented uncoordinated movements".[33]

The healing of pressure sores, another consequence of spending long periods of time in bed or in a wheelchair, is twice as fast when treated with low frequency pulsed currents. Electrical stimulation also improved healing in cases where the natural healing mechanisms of the body were not sufficient (chronic wounds, older subjects).[34, 35]

3.5   Facial Rehabilitation

This Chapter could not be finished without adding a summarised section on the treatment of Facial Paralysis, a disorder that has dramatic consequences for sufferers, who are unable to smile, laugh or even cry, have speech difficulties, eating and drinking are problematic, self esteem is often non-existent as they are aware of what they look like and how people see them, negativity abounds.

Damage to all or some axons in the facial nerve is the main cause of Facial Palsy and recovery depends on axons regrowth and muscle reinnervation, the capacity of regenerated axons to keep neuromuscular connections with the denervated facial muscles, and the muscles condition at the time of reinnervation.

Advances have also been made in studies on the positive effects of electrical stimulation on accelerating nerve regeneration after injury or disease[36] and restoring specific connections between sensory and motor axons with their respective targets.[37] It is well established that the shorter the time of denervation and the fewer axons are misdirected into inappropriate targets, the better the recovery after denervation. Electrical stimulation of activity of regenerating nerves should be beneficial for the recovery after facial palsy.

It is known that the condition of the target muscles is important for recovery of function on reinnervation. On reaching the target muscle, the nerve terminals of individual motor axons should be able to make functional contacts with as many muscle fibers as possible, so as to allow even few axons to activate a large proportion of the reinnervated muscle. In addition the muscle should be kept in a condition where even a few axons can elicit strong contractions. Moreover neuromuscular activity of immature nerve terminals during sprouting increases the motor unit territory and enhances the strength of the muscle.[38]

As more research is done into the therapeutic benefits of electrical stimulation for the treatment of Bell's palsy, there is hope that sufferers will see important improvements in their lives.

References

1. W. I. Drechsler, M. C. Cramp, and O. M. Scott, Changes in muscle strength and EMG median frequency after anterior cruciate ligament reconstruction, *Eur. J. Appl. Physiol.* **98**:613–623 (2006).
2. A. Delitto, S. J. Rose, J. M. McKowen, R. C. Lehman, J. A. Thomas, and R. A. Shively, Electrical stimulation versus voluntary exercise in strengthening thigh musculature after anterior cruciate ligament surgery, *Phys. Ther.* **68**:660–663 (1988).
3. L. Snyder-Mackler, A. Delitto, S. L. Bailey, and S. W. Stralka, Strength of the quadriceps femoris muscle and functional recovery after reconstruction of the anterior cruciate ligament. A prospective, randomized clinical trial of electrical stimulation, *J. Bone Joint Surg.* **77**:1166–1173 (1995).
4. J. E. Stevens, R. L. Mizner, and L. Snyder-Mackler, Neuromuscular electrical stimulation for quadriceps muscle strengthening after bilateral total knee arthroplasty: a case series, J. Orth. *Sports Phys. Ther.* **34**:21–29 (2004).
5. M. M. Dimitrijevic, and M. R. Dimitrijevic, Clinical elements for the neuromuscular stimulation and functional electrical stimulation protocols in the practice of neurorehabilitation, *Artif. Organs* **26**:256–259 (2002).
6. L. R. Sheffler, and J. Chae, Neuromuscular electrical stimulation in neurorehabilitation, *Muscle Nerve* **35**:562–590 (2007).
7. J. Worthington, and L. Desouza, The use of clinical measures in the evaluation of neuromuscular stimulation in multiple sclerosis patients, in: *Current Concepts in Multiple Sclerosis*, edited by H. Wielhölter, J. Dichgans, and J. Mertin (Elsevier, Amsterdam, 1991), pp. 213–218.

8. A. Kralj, and L. Vodovnik, Functional electrical stimulation of the extremities: Part 1, *J. Med. Eng. Technol.* **1**:2–15 (1971).
9. J. H. Grill, and P. H. Peckham, Functional neuromuscular stimulation for combined control of elbow extension and hand grasp in C5 and C6 quadriplegics, *IEEE Trans. Rehabil. Eng.* **6**:190–1999 (1998).
10. U. Carraro, K. Rossini, W. Mayr, and H. Kern, Muscle fiber regeneration in human permanent lower motoneuron denervation: relevance to safety and effectiveness of FES-training, which induces muscle recovery in SCI subjects, *Artif. Organs* **29**:187–191 (2005).
11. H. Kern, C. Hofer, M. Strohhofer, W. Mayr, W. Richter, and H. Stöhr, Standing up with denervated muscles in humans using functional electrical stimulation, *Artif. Organs* **23**:447–452 (1999).
12. M. Mödlin, C. Forstner, C. Hofer, W. Mayr, W. Richter, U. Carraro, F. Protasi, and H. Kern, Electrical stimulation of denervated muscles: first results of a clinical study, *Artif. Organs* **29**:203–206 (2005).
13. G. Alon, A. F. Levitt, and P. A. McCarthy, Functional electrical stimulation enhancement of upper extremity functional recovery during stroke rehabilitation: a pilot study, *Neurorehab. Neural Repair* **21**:207–215 (2007).
14. H. Kobayashi, H. Onishi, K. Ihashi, R. Yagi, and Y. Handa, Reduction in subluxation and improved muscle function of the hemiplegic shoulder joint after therapeutic electrical stimulation, *J. Electromyogr. Kinesiol* **9**:327–336 (1999).
15. C. J. Newsam, and L. L. Baker, Effect of electric stimulation facilitation program on quadriceps motor unit recruitment after stroke, *Arch. Phys. Rehab.* **85**:2040–2045 (2004).
16. T. J. Kimberley, and P. T. Carey, Neuromuscular electrical stimulation in stroke rehabilitation, *Minn. Med.* **85**:34–37 (2002).
17. W. W. Glenn, and M. L. Phelps, Diaphragm pacing by electrical stimulation of the phrenic nerve, *Neurosurgery* **17**:974–984 (1985).
18. S. Jezernik, M. Craggs, W. M. Grill, G. Creasey, and N. J. Rijkhoff, Electrical stimulation for the treatment of bladder dysfunction: current status and future possibilities, *Neurol. Res.* **24**:413–430 (2002).
19. L. Brubaker, Electrical stimulation in overactive bladder, *Urology* **55**:17–32 (2000).
20. O. M. Scott, G. Vrbová, S. A. Hyde, and V. Dubowitz, Responses of muscle of patients with Duchenne muscular atrophy to chronic electrical stimulation, *J. Neurol. Neurosurg. Psychiatr.* **49**:1427–1434 (1986).
21. O. M. Scott, S. A. Hyde, G. Vrbová, and V. Dubowitz, Therapeutic possibilities of chronic low frequency electrical stimulation in children with Duchene muscular dystrophy, *J. Neurol. Sci.* **95**:171–182 (1990).
22. A. Zupan, Long-term electrical stimulation of muscles in children with Duchene and Becker muscular dystrophy, *Muscle Nerve* **15**:362–367 (1992).
23. A. Zupan, M. Gregoric, V. Valencic, and S. Vandot, Effects of electrical stimulation on muscles of children with Duchenne and Becker muscular dystrophy, *Neuropediatrics* **24**:189–192 (1993).
24. G. Vrbová, Function induced modifications of gene expression: an alternative approach to gene therapy of Duchene muscular dystrophy, *J. Muscle Res. Cell Motil.* **25**:187–192 (2004).
25. V. A. Convertino, S. A. Bloomfield, and J. F. Greenfield, An overview of the issues: physiological effects of bed rest and restricted physical activity, *Med. Sci Sports Exerc.* **29**:187–190 (1997).
26. J. Duchateau, Bed rest induces neural and contractile adaptation in triceps surae, *Med. Sci. Sports Exerc.* **27**:1581–1589 (1995).
27. K. Takenaka, Y. Suzuki, K. Kawakubo, Y. Haruna, R. Yanagibori, H. Kashihara, T. Igarashi, F. Watanabe, M. Omata, F Bonde-Petersen, et al., Cardiovascular effects of 20 days bed rest in healthy young subjects. *Acta Physiol. Scand. Suppl* **616**:59–63 (1994).
28. G. Ferretti, G. Antonutto, C. Denis, H. Hoppeler, A. E. Minetti, M. V. Narici, and D. Desplanches, The interplay of central and peripheral factors in limiting maximal O2 consumption in man after prolonged bed rest, *J. Physiol.* **501**:677–686 (1997).
29. S. A. Bloomfied, Changes in musculoskeletal structure and function with prolonged bed rest, *Med. Sci. Sports Exerc.* **29**:197–206 (1997).

30. T. Iwasaki, N. Shiba, H. Matsuse, T. Nago, Y. Umezu, Y. Tagawa, K. Nagata, and J. R. Bassford, Improvement of knee strength through training by means of combined electrical stimulation and voluntary muscle contraction, *Tohoku J. Exp. Med.* **209**:33–40 (2006).
31. L. I. Kakurin, B. B. Yegorov, Y. I. Il'ina, and M. A. Cherepakhin, Effects of muscle electrostimulation during simulated weightlessness, *Acta Astronaut.* **2**:241–246 (1975).
32. M. A. Cherepakhin, L. I. Kakurin, E. I. Ilina–Kakueva, and G. T. Fedorenko, Evaluation of the effectiveness of electrostimulation of the muscles in preventing disorders related to prolonged limited motor activity in man, *Kosm. Biol. Aviakosm. Med.* **11**:64–68 (1977).
33. W. Mayr, M. Bijak, W. Girsch, C. Hofer, H. Lanmüller, D. Rafolt, M. Rakos, S. Sauermann, C. Schmutterer, G. Schnetz, E. Unger, and G. Freilinger, MYOSIM FES to prevent muscle atrophy in microgravity and bed rest: preliminary report, *Artif. Organs* **23**:428–431 (1999).
34. A. Stefanovska, L. Vodovnik, H. Benko, and R. N. Turk, Treatment of chronic wounds by means of electric and electromagnetic fields. Part 2. Value of FES parameters for pressure sore treatment. *Med. Biol. Eng. Comput.* **31**:213–220 (1993).
35. K. M. Bogie, S. I. Reger, S. P. Levine, and V. Saghal, Electrical stimulation for pressure sore prevention and wound healing, *Assist. Technol.* **12**:50–66 (2000).
36. A. A. Al Majeed, T. M. Brushart, and T. Gordon, Electrical stimulation accelerates and increases expression of BDNF and trkB mRNA in regenerating rat femoral motoneurones, *Eur. J. Neurosci.* **12**:4381–4390 (2000).
37. T. M. Brushart, R. Jari, V. Verge, C. Rohde, and T. Gordon, Electrical stimulation restores the specificity of sensory axon regeneration, *Exp. Neurol.* **194**:221–229 (2005).
38. G. Vrbová, Rationale for activating nerves and muscles in patients with facial palsy with appropriate patterns of activity, 2001 May, Dept of Anatomy and Developmental Biology, University College London (2001).
39. K. M. Bogie, and R. J. Triolo, Effects of regular use of neuromuscular electrical stimulation on tissue health, *J. Rehabil. Res. Dev.* **40**:469–475 (2003).
40. R. B. Stein, T. Gordon, J. Jefferson, A. Shafterberger, J. F. Yang, J. T. de Zepetnek, and M. Belanger, Optimal stimulation of paralyzed muscle after spinal cord injury, *J. Appl. Physiol.* **72**:1392–1400 (1992).
41. T. P. Martin, R. B. Stein, P. H. Hoeppner, and D. C. Reid, Influence of electrical stimulation on the morphological and metabolic properties of paralyzed muscle, *J. Appl. Physiol.* **72**:1401–1406 (1992).
42. R. M. Crameri, A. Weston, M. Climstein, G. M. Davis, and J. R. Sutton, Effects of electrical stimulation-induced leg training on skeletal muscle adaptability in spinal cord injury, *Scand. J. Med. Sci. Sports* **12**:316–322 (2003).
43. P. D. Faghri, and J. Yount, Electrically induced and voluntary activation of physiologic muscle pump: a comparison between spinal cord-injured and able-bodied individuals, *Clin. Rehabil.* **16**:878–888 (2002).
44. R. T. Katz, D. Green, T. Sullivan, and G. Yarkony, Functional electric stimulation to enhance systemic fibinolytic activity in spinal cord injury patients, *Arch. Phys. Med. Rehabil.* **68**:423–416 (1987).
45. D. H. Thijssen, P. Heesterbeek, D. J. van Kuppevelt, J. Duysens, and M. T. Hopman, Local vascular adaptation after hybrid training in spinal cord-injured subjects, *Med. Sci. Sports Exerc.* **37**:1112–1118 (2005).
46. I. Arvidsson, H. Arvidsson, E. Eriksson, and E. Jansson, Prevention of quadriceps wasting after immobilization: an evaluation of the effect of electrical stimulation, *Orthopedics* **9**:1519–1528 (1986).
47. N. Gould, D. Donnermeyer, G. G. Gammon, M. Popez, and T. Ashikaga, Transcutanous muscle stimulation to retard disuse atrophy after open meniscotomy, *Clin. Orthoped. Rel. Res.* **17**:180–195 (1983).
48. M. R. Duvoisin, V. A. Convertino, P. Buchanan, P. D. Gollnick, and G. A. Dudely, Characteristics and preliminary observations of the influence of elctromyostimulation on the size and function of human skeletal muscle during 30 days of simulated microgravity, *Aviat. Space Environ. Med.* **60**:671–678 (1989).

Chapter 4
Electrical Stimulation for Health, Beauty, Fitness, Sports Training and Rehabilitation

A Users Guide

Kristin Schaefer Centofanti

Abstract With the development of modern electronics, electrical stimulation has become a widely accepted therapeutic tool for muscle rehabilitation and recovery. However the scientific and medical communities have tended to sideline or dismiss the use of electrotherapy for healthy muscles. This chapter covers the various applications and benefits of electrical stimulation on normal healthy individuals for toning, strengthening, body shaping and general fitness. This section also offers practical protocols for both the training of healthy muscles and the recovery or improvement of muscles and tissues that have been damaged or are diseased.

Keywords Biphasic, body shaping, electrode pads, electrotherapy, frequency, intensity, motor point, motor unit, pad layout, pulse width, pulses per second, ramp time, TENS, waveform

4.1 The Use of Electrical Stimulation

4.1.1 Electrical Stimulation Devices

When looking at Electrical Stimulation (sometimes known as ES, or EMS, or NMES) and its applications, a primary focus must inevitably be on the development of reliable and readily available machines that can deliver biologically appropriate impulses to living tissue. Since the 1950s, with the emergence of mass produced circuit boards and battery controlled devices, a variety of systems have not only been made available to research scientists, doctors and therapists, but also to the general consumer.

Indeed, the launch of one of the very first commercially available battery operated stimulators for the general public was in the UK.[1] The small four channel units were safe, portable battery operated systems that used carbon graphite embedded in rubber pads (electrodes) as a way to conduct the signal safely. The operating instructions were simple and designed for individual home use as a method for figure control and body shaping.

JKC Research Partnership, London E5 8AP, UK

G. Vrbová et al., *Application of Muscle/Nerve Stimulation in Health and Disease*,
© Springer Science + Business Media B.V. 2008

As a consequence, electrical stimulation entered the world of the consumer before being generally used or accepted by the majority of the scientific research community. This has been both a help and a hindrance to the development of electrical stimulation. On the one hand, good market potential for stimulation devices has assured a steady flow of high quality and reasonably priced machines that offer more and more sophisticated and safe applications. On the other hand, the scientific community has perhaps viewed electrical stimulation with a certain amount of disdain and suspicion, as some health and figure shaping benefits have been over emphasized to maximize the selling potential of these machines in a highly competitive market. We are in the unusual position of having a vast choice of stimulators available to us, both for therapists and home users, yet the question "does it really work" is still uppermost in many people's mind.

4.1.2   Exercise and Dieting

Barely less than 50 years ago, the standard medical opinion was that only strictly controlled dieting would lead to weight and inch loss. It was believed that active exercise consumed calories only temporarily, with the metabolism returning to normal once the physical effort had stopped. With the emergence of a sedentary society, doctors then began to understand the true relationship between lack of exercise and weight gain. They observed the long term and cumulative benefits of exercise: once muscles are activated, a combination of physiological processes takes place and keeps on working long after the physical movement has stopped. Nowadays most people are aware of the value of exercise and how important a role it plays in weight and body shape control, as well as the importance of keeping healthy muscles toned up and maintaining fitness levels. This has all become common knowledge.

But how should one exercise? Does a physical activity have to be exhausting to be beneficial? Is crash exercising as harmful potentially as crash dieting? Is there any other way?

It is at this juncture that the benefits of electrical stimulation become apparent, as it provides a safe, fast and effective method for exercising and toning muscles, thus shaping the body and keeping it active.[2–10] Does this mean that electrical stimulation replaces active exercise? No, on the contrary, what it does imply is that if a person tones his/her muscles with electrical stimulation, afterwards that person is more likely to participate in sporting activities as the body is ready, fit, willing and able to take on physical activity. Thus electrical stimulation can actually *lead* to exercise.

4.1.3   Concentrating the Benefits

As we have seen in the chapter about muscle plasticity, with electrical stimulation "all motor units in the muscles (i.e., even those normally not recruited in exercise) can be simultaneously activated by the same pattern of activity."[11] With ordinary exercise the muscles are recruited in a set hierarchical way; the small motor units are activated first and only very progressively and after much effort are the large body shaping muscles brought into action. Thus it can take up to half an hour of vigorous active training to reach the muscles one wants to work on, and, unless the training is intense and regular, the body shaping results can be minimal. With electrical stimulation, preset pulses in varying sequences can reach those muscles in seconds, faster than with ordinary exercise; in fact it is the large motor units that tend to respond first at low current intensity.[11]

In their 1999 study, Drs Pete and Vrbová state: "electrical stimulation can attain much higher levels of activity over time than any exercise regime and, therefore, the adaptive potential of the system is challenged to its limits".[11] They go on further to explain that "high levels of activity can be imposed on the target muscle by electrical stimulation from the beginning, because the central nervous, cardiovascular, and other systems will not interfere with and limit the amount of activity, as is the case in exercise."

Thus electrical stimulation of healthy muscles can be used in conjunction with exercise, as a way of enhancing the results of activity; as a form of preparation for a sport, like football or ski, for example, which can be hard on an unprepared body; or as a supplement to exercise when age or sedentary habits created by modern lifestyles set in and allow muscles to deteriorate.[10]

The fact that specific muscle groups can be individually targeted, without effort, in a concentrated manner unequalled by physical effort and that the protocols of electrical stimulation can be specifically arranged in different sequences or patterns suitable for a particular objective, makes ES a very useful tool for reaching the muscles that shape the body and face. Whether the aim is fitness or appearance, strength or stamina, all are human needs and ES represents a human solution for our times and for the future.

Paradoxically, it is this 'unnatural' form of generating muscle activity (electrical stimulation) that has made it possible to study and understand the way muscles work and how to reach them.

More in depth explanations of muscle properties and functions, how Electrical Stimulation affects them and in turn how muscle activity helps to shape the body, restore strength and stamina, aid recovery and rehabilitation, deal with injuries and disease as well as improve fitness, are covered in previous chapters. Once these principles of how an electrical signal affects the body and the plasticity of muscles are understood, both the home user and the specialized therapists will be able to operate these stimulators with realistic expectations and thus obtain optimum and reliable results.

This section deals specifically with the practical application and suggested protocols for use on normal healthy muscles as well as injured or diseased muscles.

4.2   Stimulation Parameters

Establishing the best waveform, an appropriate pulse width, the right frequency, the correct stimulation and pause time are an essential part of electrotherapy treatments. The following protocols have been devised by using models based on active exercise regimes combined with our present understanding of how electrical impulses affect the body. We can thus make a muscle work quickly, slowly, vigorously or gently etc. as if it were undergoing voluntary exercise and we also take into account the way electrical impulses by pass the normal communication processes and stimulate tissue directly.

4.2.1 Basic Terminology

- **Waveform:** the shape of an individual impulse. The proliferation of commercially available stimulators means that a variety of waveforms are offered and it is often difficult to understand which signal is the most appropriate for therapeutic use. Fortunately, an easy and general guideline is **comfort**. This is normally achieved when the impulse reaches its peak rise time quickly.[12] In more modern machinery there is also a choice between a mono-phasic and bi-phasic waveform. A mono-phasic waveform current flows asymmetrically from the negative pad to the positive pad; it can be perceived as smoother and more comfortable with the negative electrode giving a slightly stronger stimulation. A bi-phasic waveform has the current flowing in either direction and thus it has no negative or positive pole. It is sometimes perceived as a sharper sensation, therefore many machines deliver a mono-phasic waveform so that a stronger intensity can be comfortably applied. The other advantage of a mono-phasic system is the use of the negative electrode for areas that need more stimulation and the use of the weaker positive electrode for areas that are more sensitive, although this does not mean that biphasic waveforms cannot be used effectively.

- **Frequency:** this is the number of pulses per second (pps) and is measured in Hertz (i.e. 40 Hz would mean a frequency of 40 pulses per second). As has been pointed out in this book, along with other supporting research, changing the pulses per second affects the tissues differently.[6–16] Man and colleagues[17] established that there is likely to be considerable subject variation in response to electrical stimulation and optimization may relate more to the subject than the stimulation parameters themselves, but the generally accepted stimulation parameters for human skeletal muscles is 1–100 Hz. As a general guideline low frequency stimulation of 10–25 Hz is best to encourage slow muscle fibre activity, whereas 45–75 Hz will encourage fast muscle fibre activity.[4–7] Frequencies between 1 and 10 Hz are used for pain suppression, endorphin release and tissue repair, 75–100 Hz for improved circulation and gate transcutaneous electrical nerve stimulation (TENS) pain suppression.[18–20]

- **Pulse width:** this is the time each individual pulse is on (pulse duration) and is measured in microseconds. Widening or narrowing the pulse width can alter the depth of the current penetration and also specifically alter the amount of electricity reaching the body tissues without increasing or decreasing the overall intensity.

- **Stimulation time** (sometimes referred to as contraction time): this is the total time a sequence of pulses is on and is usually measured in seconds or parts of a second. It is also called a stimulation envelope as it groups a series of impulses.

- **Pause time** (sometimes referred to as relaxation time): this is the time when the stimulation is off.

- **Ramp time:** this is an electrical inhibition which ensures the smooth and gradual delivery of a stimulation envelope (group of impulses) and is usually measured in seconds or parts of a second.

4.3   Applying Electrical Stimulation to the Body

There are now many accepted uses for electrical applications: muscle toning,[10] strengthening and shaping, figure control,[2–9] increasing blood flow,[12,21] pain relief,[22,23] tissue regeneration,[24–26] oedema reduction[27] and dermal repair,[28–30] to name but a few.

It is important to know which are the best positions for electrode placement when using electrical stimulation in its different applications. Generally, either the origin or insertion of a muscle or its motor point is used for placement as the pumping action of the muscles enhances the desired effect, but in certain cases the electrodes will be placed directly over the area that needs treating. In this case no muscular movement is either seen or felt.

In order to optimize the functional aspect of electrical stimulation via the muscles, it is extremely useful to be familiar with the location of skeletal muscles and their corresponding motor points.

4.3.1   Mapping the Motor Points of Human Skeletal Muscles

A motor point is the area of skin overlying the muscle at which the smallest amount of currents activates this muscle. It is closest to were the motor nerve trumk enteres the muscle, usually over the belly of each muscle. (Large muscle may have more than one motor point).[19] The following diagrams (Figs. 4.1–4.3) are a useful guide

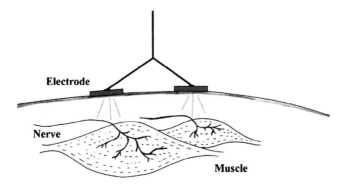

Fig. 4.1 Muscle motor point

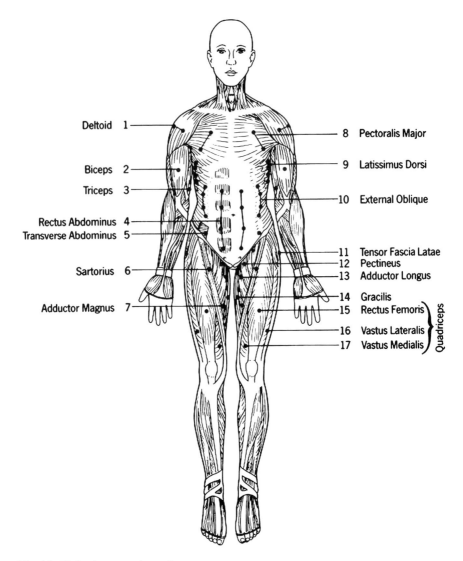

Fig. 4.2 Skeletal motor points – front

to locate the trigger points for the major body shaping muscles. As a general rule, electrodes are placed over these motor points to directly stimulate one or more muscle groups. If the electrodes are placed accurately then the stimulation sensation is smooth, comfortable and easily tolerated. This means one can therefore increase the intensity sufficiently to obtain good muscular contractions for fast and reliable results.

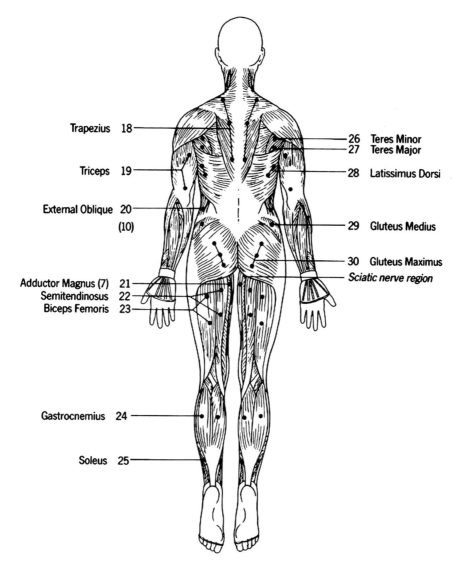

Fig. 4.3 Skeletal motor points – back

4.4 Protocols and Electrode Pad Placements

4.4.1 Stimulation Parameters

With each set of pad placement suggestions (Figs. 4.4–4.8) there are also stimulation parameter suggestions (Tables 4.1 and 4.2) which are based on empirical observation of results and the information gathered regarding the effects of different

Fig. 4.4 Abdominal pad layout small frame

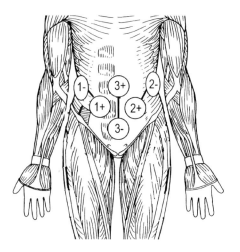

Fig. 4.5 Buttocks pad layout small frame

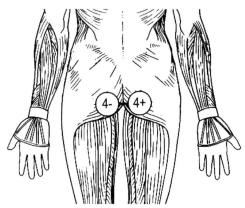

Fig. 4.6 Waist pad layout

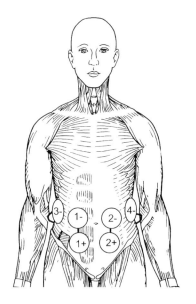

Fig. 4.7 Waist pad layout back view

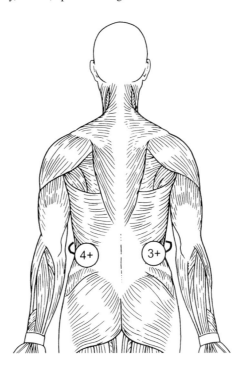

Fig. 4.8 Abdominal layout large frame. Suitable for stimulators with at least 10 outlets (20 electrode pads).

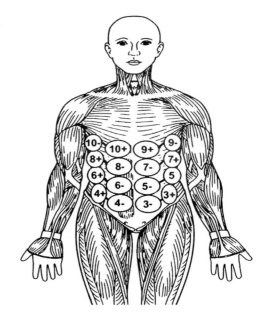

frequencies, pulse widths, stimulation times and how the body responds generally to physical activity.

These parameters are also gender specific in many cases as the differences between male and female anatomy, such as muscle mass, fat and skin resistance, are relevant to the application of electrical stimulation.

Generally, electrical stimulation can be applied every other day, sometimes once a day with high quality stimulators which deliver a comfortable and easily tolerated signal. Some body shaping results can be expected after 3–6 sessions. Normally 12–21 sessions are required to achieve good results.

Some stimulators do not allow you to change the pulse width or ramp time. In this case simply adjust the stimulation time, pause time and frequency to approximate the protocol parameters.

In the electrode placements that follow, a positive and negative layout has been used to take account of a monophasic type current where the negative electrode is slightly stronger than the positive electrode. If a biphasic waveform is used, the current will alternate from positive to negative, therefore the polarity of the electrodes will no longer matter.

When using a monophasic current it is important to place the negative pad on the area that needs the stronger stimulation and the positive pad on the more sensitive area so that optimum and comfortable treatments are obtained.

4.4.2 Usage

Generally three sessions per week, over a period of 4–6 weeks, gives good initial results depending on the body shaping, toning, sports training or rehabilitation and recovery needs.

In the case of obese users, a daily stimulation may be required with sessions of up to 1 hour as the externally applied signal will have difficulty penetrating thick layers of fat.

It is ideal of course to also follow a healthy eating plan when embarking on a course of stimulation sessions in order to maximize the health enhancing benefits and accelerate the body shaping results whilst losing weight.

Once good results have been obtained the sessions may be reduced to once or twice a week until the user feels that optimum body shaping has been achieved.

As mentioned before, one of the questions most often repeated at this stage is "does using regular electrical stimulation replace active exercise?"

In fact the reverse is true as in most cases the use of electrical stimulation encourages people to do more active exercise not less. The effortless relaxing application of specific signals to tone, shape and strengthen the body has the inevitable effect of giving people the confidence and energy to lead a more physically active life as the electrically trained muscles respond more readily. Thus a sporting or physically demanding leisure activity, which may have been avoided in the past due to an overly sedentary lifestyle, will no longer be seen as a chore but as an attractive pastime as the body will be more willing and able to respond.

4.4.3 Electrode Pads

The figures that follow will indicate suggested placement layouts of electrodes. Commercially available electrodes come in a variety of shapes and materials.

Re-useable electrodes are normally carbon graphite. They need to be thoroughly immersed in water so that there is adequate conductivity in order for the impulses to penetrate the skin and give a comfortable effective stimulation. They will also need to be held in place by stretch straps of differing lengths to accommodate various body areas.

Self adhesive electrodes are also available and are extremely practical as a coating of sticky conductive gel is used on top of a wire mesh or thin flexible carbon pad, thus eliminating the need for water or straps.

In the figures illustrated, the electrode shape is round with a pad diameter of approximately 7 cm for body stimulation and 2.5 cm for the face.

There are also square, rectangular and oval electrodes of varying sizes commercially available.

The essential element to remember when selecting an electrode is the purpose of its application. A smaller electrode will send the impulse to a narrow specific area, whereas a larger electrode will diffuse the signal over a wider area, making it generally more comfortable and easier to reach motor points.

A 7 cm diameter or square electrode for body stimulation and a 2.5 cm circle for face has empirically been shown to be the best combination of size versus comfort for general electrical stimulation use.

4.4.4 Index of Pad Placements

BODY SHAPING AND TONING

1. Abdomen/Waist Stimulation
2. Buttocks and Hips Stimulation
3. Thigh Stimulation
4. Bust/Pectoral Stimulation
5. Arms Stimulation
6. Calves/Ankle Stimulation
7. Posture
8. Facial Stimulation

SPORTS TRAINING

1. Abdomen Stimulation
2. Quadriceps Stimulation
3. Gluteus and Hamstring Stimulation
4. Pectorals, Biceps and Triceps Stimulation
5. Gastrocnemius Stimulation
6. Whole Body Stimulation

INCREASING RANGE OF MOTION
TENS
REPAIR, RECOVERY AND REHABILITATION

4.5 Body Shaping and Toning

The following protocols and pad placements are suitable for normal healthy people who wish to tone and shape their body to obtain a more attractive silhouette and to enhance general fitness levels.

4.5.1 Abdominal Stimulation

When stimulating the Abdomen it is always useful to also stimulate Buttocks as well, when possible, as the muscles work together to shape the trunk and re-align the silhouette (see Figs. 4.4–4.10 and Tables 4.1 and 4.2).

Table 4.1 Abdominal stimulation parameters – female – total time 45 minutes

Phase	1	2	3	4	5	6	7
Time in minutes	5	5	10	8	7	8	2
Stimulation in seconds	2	4	8	10	6	4	1.2
Pause in seconds	2.5	4	6	1	4	4	0.5
Frequency (Hz)	90	50	10	4	30	65	100
Pulse width in microseconds	200	300	500	600	360	300	80
Ramp in seconds	0.5	0.5	0.9	1.3	0.6	0.5	0.2

Table 4.2 Abdominal stimulation parameters – male – total time 40 minutes

Phase	1	2	3	4	5	6	7
Time in minutes	5	10	5	5	8	5	2
Stimulation in seconds	2	4	8	10	6	4	1.2
Pause in seconds	2.5	4	6	1	4	4	0.5
Frequency (Hz)	90	60	10	4	45	65	100
Pulse width in microseconds	260	360	600	700	400	360	90
Ramp in seconds	0.5	0.5	0.9	1.3	0.6	0.5	0.2

Phase 1 – preparation: Turn up the stimulation gradually, until a gentle pulsed tingling is felt, then increase the intensity until a fast pumping is felt.

Phases 2 to 6 – activation: Increase the intensity until a strong visible movement is seen and felt.

Phase 7 – cool down: Turn down the intensity gradually until a mild tingling pulse is felt. Pad placement suitable for stimulators with at least 4 outlets (8 electrode pads).

For medium to small frame bodies with stimulators that have 8 electrode pads, a pair of electrode pads may be placed on the buttocks also, as this will tense the gluteal muscles along with the abdominal muscles and force the pelvis to tilt into a correct postural position thus flattening the tummy and improving the postural stance.

Note: the negative (slightly stronger) pad has been placed on the left buttock as most right handed people have a faster stimulation response on their right side, thus the slightly weaker positive pad will give a good response whereas the weaker left side will generally benefit from the stronger impulse of the negative electrode pad. For left handed people you may wish to reverse the negative and positive pad placement to balance the stimulation effect.

Pad placement suitable for stimulators with at least 4 outlets (8 electrode pads).

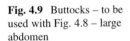

Fig. 4.9 Buttocks – to be used with Fig. 4.8 – large abdomen

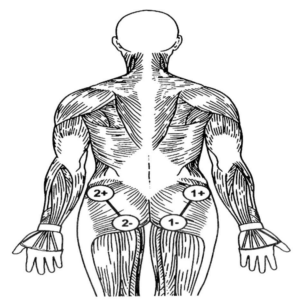

4.5.2 Buttocks and Hips Stimulation

Phase 1 – preparation: Turn up the stimulation gradually, until an intermittent tingling is felt, then increase the intensity until a gentle pumping is felt.

Phases 2 to 6 – activation: Increase the intensity until a strong, smooth, visible movement is seen and felt.

Phase 7 – cool down: Turn down the intensity gradually until a mild tingling pulse is felt.

Pad placement suitable for stimulators with at least 6 outlets (12 electrode pads). (see Fig. 4.10 and Tables 4.3 and 4.4)

Fig. 4.10 Buttocks & hips pad layout

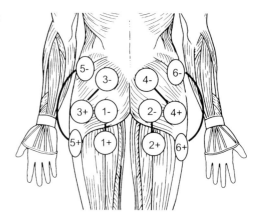

Table 4.3 Buttocks & hips parameters – female – total time 30 minutes

Phase	1	2	3	4	5	6	7
Time in minutes	5	5	5	5	5	3	2
Stimulation in seconds	3	6	8	4	3	5	1.2
Pause in seconds	2	5	4	4	4	5	0.5
Frequency (Hz)	100	65	10	50	75	45	100
Pulse width in microseconds	200	300	500	300	260	260	80
Ramp in seconds	0.5	0.7	0.9	0.5	0.5	0.5	0.2

Table 4.4 Buttocks & hips parameters – male – total time 30 minutes

Phase	1	2	3	4	5	6	7
Time in minutes	5	5	5	5	5	3	2
Stimulation in seconds	4	6	8	4	3	5	1.2
Pause in seconds	3	4	4	4	4	5	0.5
Frequency (Hz)	100	65	10	50	75	45	100
Pulse width in microseconds	300	400	600	340	300	300	90
Ramp in seconds	0.5	0.7	0.9	0.5	0.5	0.5	0.2

4.5.3   Thigh Stimulation

Phase 1 – preparation: Turn up the stimulation gradually, until an intermittent tingling is felt, then increase the intensity until a gentle pumping is felt.

Phases 2 to 6 – activation: Increase the intensity until a strong, smooth, visible movement is seen and felt.

Phase 7 - cool down: Turn down the intensity gradually until a mild tingling pulse is felt.

Pad placement suitable for stimulators with at least 4 outlets (8 electrode pads) (Figs 4.11 and Table 4.5 and 4.6).

Fig. 4.11 Inner & outer thigh pad layout 1

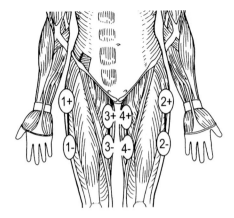

Table 4.5 Thigh stimulation parameters – female – total time 30 minutes

Phase	1	2	3	4	5	6	7
Time in minutes	5	5	5	5	5	3	2
Stimulation in seconds	5	3	1	10	6	4	1.2
Pause in seconds	4	4	0.7	1	4	4	0.5
Frequency (Hz)	10	65	100	4	45	8	100
Pulse width in microseconds	400	300	260	500	360	500	80
Ramp in seconds	0.9	0.5	0.3	0.9	0.6	0.5	0.2

Table 4.6 Thigh stimulation – male – total time 30 minutes

Phase	1	2	3	4	5	6	7
Time in minutes	5	5	5	5	5	3	2
Stimulation in seconds	6	4	1.5	10	6	4	1.2
Pause in seconds	3	4	0.8	1	4	4	0.5
Frequency (Hz)	10	60	10	6	50	8	100
Pulse width in microseconds	500	360	500	600	360	600	90
Ramp in seconds	0.3	0.5	1.3	0.9	0.6	0.5	0.2

Pad placement suitable for stimulators with at least 6 outlets (12 electrode pads) (Fig. 4.12 and Tables 4.5 and 4.6).

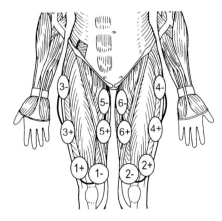

Fig. 4.12 Inner & outer thigh pad layout 2

4.5.4   Bust/Pectorals Stimulation

Phase 1 – preparation: Turn up the stimulation gradually, until an intermittent tingling is felt, then increase the intensity until a gentle pumping is felt.

Phases 2, 5 & 6 activation: Increase the intensity until a smooth, comfortable movement is seen and felt. The stimulation should not be too strong.

Phases 3 & 4 detox: Decrease the intensity until a mild pumping is felt.

Phase 7 – cool down: Turn down the intensity gradually until a mild tingling pulse is felt (Figs. 4.13 and 4.14, Tables 4.5 and 4.6).

Pad placement suitable for stimulators with at least 4 outlets (8 electrode pads).

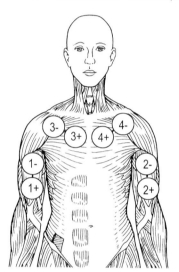

Fig. 4.13 Bust/pectoral pad layout

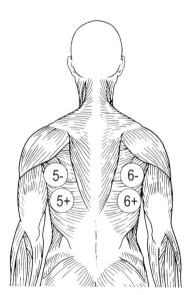

Fig. 4.14 Bra strap pad layout

Table 4.7 Bust/pectorals stimulation parameters female – total time 30 minutes

Phase	1	2	3	4	5	6	7
Time in minutes	5	5	5	5	5	3	2
Stimulation in seconds	3	3	5	1	4	6	2
Pause in seconds	3	2.5	3	0.3	4.5	6	0.5
Frequency (Hz)	90	60	10	4	45	65	90
Pulse width in microseconds	150	150	220	300	200	200	80
Ramp in seconds	0.3	0.5	1.3	0.9	0.6	0.5	0.2

Table 4.8 Bust/pectorals stimulation parameters male – total time 30 minutes

Phase	1	2	3	4	5	6	7
Time in minutes	5	5	5	5	5	3	2
Stimulation in seconds	2	4	8	10	6	4	1.2
Pause in seconds	2.5	4	6	1	4	4	0.5
Frequency (Hz)	90	60	10	4	45	65	100
Pulse width in microseconds	200	200	260	300	220	220	80
Ramp in seconds	0.3	0.5	1.3	0.9	0.6	0.5	0.2

This layout is designed for women who have sagging muscles and a build up of fat around the bra strap area. It is to be used in conjunction with Fig. 4.13 bust/pectoral layout.

4.5.5 Arms Stimulation

Phase 1 – preparation: Turn up the stimulation gradually, until an intermittent tingling is felt, then increase the intensity until a gentle pumping is felt.

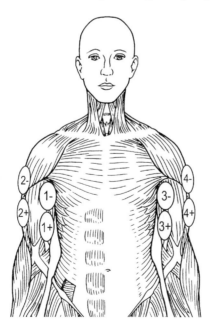

Fig. 4.15 Arms layout

Table 4.9 Arms stimulation parameters female – total time 30 minutes

Phase	1	2	3	4	5	6	7
Time in minutes	5	5	5	5	5	3	2
Stimulation in seconds	3	4	8	4	6	4	1.2
Pause in seconds	2.5	4	6	2	2	4	0.5
Frequency (Hz)	90	60	10	65	4	65	100
Pulse width in microseconds	220	220	300	200	300	200	80
Ramp in seconds	0.3	0.5	1.3	0.5	0.6	0.5	0.2

Table 4.10 Arms stimulation parameters male – total time 30 minutes

Phase	1	2	3	4	5	6	7
Time in minutes	5	5	5	5	5	3	2
Stimulation in seconds	4	4	6	10	6	4	1.2
Pause in seconds	2.5	3	3	8	4	4	0.5
Frequency (Hz)	70	60	10	50	10	65	100
Pulse width in microseconds	200	200	300	220	300	220	80
Ramp in seconds	0.3	0.5	0.9	0.9	0.6	0.5	0.2

Phases 2 to 6 activation: Increase the intensity until a smooth, comfortable movement is seen and felt. The stimulation should be very vigorous but not uncomfortable.

Phase 7 – cool down: Turn down the intensity gradually until a mild tingling pulse is felt.

Pad placement suitable for stimulators with at least 4 outlets (8 electrode pads) (Fig. 4.15 and Tables 4.9 and 4.10).

4.5.6 *Calves/Ankles Stimulation*

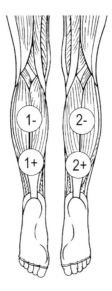

Fig. 4.16 Calves layout

Table 4.11 Calves & ankles stimulation parameters female – total time 30 minutes

Phase	1	2	3	4	5	6	7
Time in minutes	5	5	5	5	5	3	2
Stimulation in seconds	1	4	3	6	8	4	1.2
Pause in seconds	1	4	3.5	4	4	4	0.5
Frequency (Hz)	100	40	50	10	4	25	100
Pulse width in microseconds	200	220	200	300	300	220	80
Ramp in seconds	0.3	0.5	0.5	0.5	0.9	0.5	0.2

Table 4.12 Calves & ankles stimulation parameters male – total time 30 minutes

Phase	1	2	3	4	5	6	7
Time in minutes	5	5	5	5	5	3	2
Stimulation in seconds	1	5	4	6	8	4	1.2
Pause in seconds	1	4	3.5	4	4	4	0.5
Frequency (Hz)	90	40	50	10	4	25	100
Pulse width in microseconds	260	300	300	400	400	300	80
Ramp in seconds	0.3	0.5	0.5	0.5	0.9	0.5	0.2

Phase 1 – preparation: Turn up the stimulation gradually, until an intermittent tingling is felt, then increase the intensity until a gentle pumping is felt.

Phases 2, 3 & 6 activation: Increase the intensity until a smooth, comfortable movement is seen and felt. The stimulation should not be too strong.

Phases 4 & 5 detox: Decrease the intensity until a mild pumping is felt.

Phase 7 – cool down: Turn down the intensity gradually until a mild tingling pulse is felt.

Pad placement suitable for stimulators with at least 2 outlets (4 electrode pads) (Fig. 4.16 and Tables 4.11 and 4.12).

Pad placement suitable for stimulators with at least 4 outlets (8 electrode pads) (Fig. 4.17).

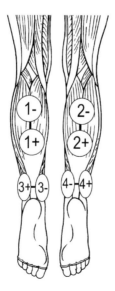

Fig. 4.17 Calves & ankles layout

4.5.7 Posture

Apart from lack of exercise which leads to flaccid muscles, poor posture is also a contributing factor to a flabby drooping appearance. The importance of a good posture is a major element for effective body shaping. Not only will ES improve the

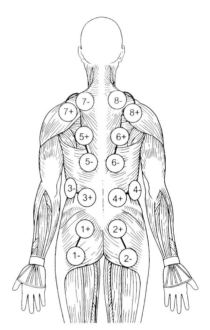

Fig. 4.18 Posture layout – back

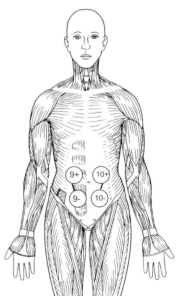

Fig. 4.19 Posture layout – abdominal – to be used in conjunction with Fig. 4.18

Table 4.13 Posture stimulation parameters female – total time 30 minutes

Phase	1	2	3	4	5	6	7
Time in minutes	2	5	5	5	5	5	3
Stimulation in seconds	10	5	4	6	3	4	1.2
Pause in seconds	1	4	3.5	4	3.5	2	0.5
Frequency (Hz)	100	10	50	4	40	4	100
Pulse width in microseconds	140	220	140	220	140	240	80
Ramp in seconds	1.2	0.5	0.5	0.5	0.5	0.5	0.2

Table 4.14 Posture stimulation parameters male – total time 30 minutes

Phase	1	2	3	4	5	6	7
Time in minutes	2	5	5	5	5	5	3
Stimulation in seconds	10	5	4	6	3	4	1.2
Pause in seconds	1	4	3.5	4	3.5	2	0.5
Frequency (Hz)	100	10	50	4	40	4	100
Pulse width in microseconds	180	280	140	220	180	240	80
Ramp in seconds	1.2	0.5	0.5	0.5	0.5	0.5	0.2

silhouette but it will also relieve some aches and pains which are caused by postural problems.

Although strong back muscles and relaxed shoulder muscles are seen as key elements for a good posture, the abdominal and gluteus muscles actually play an essential role in figure control.

Phase 1 – preparation: Turn up the stimulation gradually, until an intermittent tingling is felt.

Phases 2 to 6: Increase the intensity until a very gentle pumping is felt under the pads placed on the back and a smooth tensing is felt under the abdominal pads. The stimulation should be comfortable and relaxing at all times.

Phase 7 – cool down: Turn down the intensity gradually until only a mild tingling pulse is felt.

Pad placement suitable for stimulators with at least 10 outlets (20 electrode pads) (Figs. 4.18 and 4.19 and Tables 4.13 and 4.14).

For stimulators with fewer outlets, split the stimulation into different sessions, grouping pad layouts 1, 2, 9 & 10 in one session, then layout 5, 6, 7 & 8 in another session and layouts 3, 4, 9 & 10 in another session.

This repeats the abdominal stimulation which is key to obtaining good posture results.

4.5.8 Facial Stimulation

In the quest for a youthful appearance, facial muscles and skin may also be stimulated to improve circulation, help activate fibroblasts which produce collagen and elastin and also tone flaccid and sagging face muscles.[31–34]

Phase 1 – preparation: Turn up the stimulation gradually, until an intermittent tingling is felt.

Phases 2 to 6: Increase the intensity until a very smooth tensing is felt under the pads, there should be little visible movement. The stimulation should be comfortable and relaxing at all times.

Phase 7 – cool down: Turn down the intensity gradually until only a mild tingling pulse is felt.

Pad placement suitable for stimulators with at least 6 outlets (12 electrode pads) (Fig. 4.20 and Tables 4.15 and 4.16).

For stimulators with fewer outlets split the stimulation into different sessions, grouping 2 pairs of pad layouts and repeating the stimulation for areas that need the most lifting and toning.

A female face illustration has been used as these treatments have largely been feminine in the past, but the pad placements are also suitable for men as the facial muscles shown in part of the diagram will be suitable for both male and female.

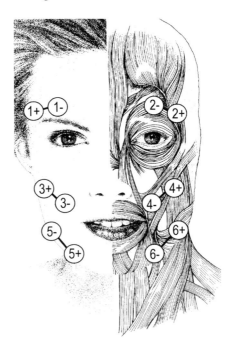

Fig. 4.20 Facial stimulation

Table 4.15 Facial stimulation parameters female – total time 15 minutes

Phase	1	2	3	4	5	6	7
Time in minutes	2	3	2	2	2	2	2
Stimulation in seconds	2	4	3	6	3	4	1.2
Pause in seconds	2.5	4	3.5	4	3.5	2	0.3
Frequency (Hz)	100	10	50	4	40	4	100
Pulse width in microseconds	140	200	140	220	140	220	80
Ramp in seconds	0.5	0.5	0.5	0.5	0.5	0.5	0.2

Table 4.16 Facial stimulation parameters male – total time 15 minutes

Phase	1	2	3	4	5	6	7
Time in minutes	2	3	2	2	2	2	2
Stimulation in seconds	2	4	3	4	3	4	2
Pause in seconds	2.5	4	3.5	4	3.5	2	0.5
Frequency (Hz)	80	10	50	4	40	4	100
Pulse width in microseconds	140	220	140	220	140	240	80
Ramp in seconds	0.5	0.5	0.5	0.5	0.5	0.5	0.2

4.6 Sports Training

These protocols and parameters have been devised to help sports people train and strengthen their muscles, whether they compete professionally or simply enjoy sports for leisure. The advantage of training with electrical stimulation is that it allows the body to activate muscles without strain or stress on load bearing joints, thus minimising the risk of injury.

4.6.1 Abdominal Stimulation

Phase 1 – preparation: Turn up the stimulation gradually, until an intermittent tingling is felt, then increase the intensity until a gentle pumping is felt.

　Phases 2 to 6 – activation: Increase the intensity until a very strong, smooth, visible movement is seen and felt.

　Phase 7 – cool down: Turn down the intensity gradually until a mild tingling pulse is felt. Pad placement suitable for stimulators with at least 4 outlets (8 electrode pads) (Fig. 4.21 and Table 4.17 and 4.18).

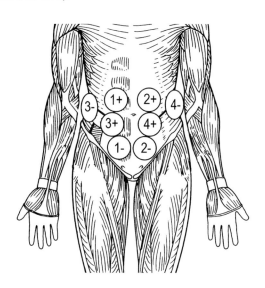

Fig. 4.21 Abdominal pad layout for sports training

Table 4.17 Abdominal training parameters female – total time 30 minutes

Phase	1	2	3	4	5	6	7
Time in minutes	5	5	5	5	5	3	2
Stimulation in seconds	4	6	1	10	4	8	2
Pause in seconds	3	4	0.5	4	3.5	3	0.5
Frequency (Hz)	80	60	50	10	40	10	100
Pulse width in microseconds	300	340	300	400	300	400	80
Ramp in seconds	0.5	0.5	0.5	0.5	0.5	0.5	0.2

Table 4.18 Abdominal training parameters male – total time 30 minutes

Phase	1	2	3	4	5	6	7
Time in minutes	5	5	5	5	5	3	2
Stimulation in seconds	4	6	1	10	4	8	2
Pause in seconds	3	4	0.5	4	3.5	3	0.5
Frequency (Hz)	80	60	50	10	40	10	100
Pulse width in microseconds	300	340	300	400	300	400	80
Ramp in seconds	0.5	0.5	0.5	0.5	0.5	0.5	0.2

4.6.2 Quadriceps Stimulation

Phase 1 – preparation: Turn up the stimulation gradually, until an intermittent tingling is felt, then increase the intensity until a gentle pumping is felt.

Phases 2 to 6 – activation: Increase the intensity until a very strong, smooth, visible movement is seen and felt.

Phase 7 – cool down: Turn down the intensity gradually until a mild tingling pulse is felt. Pad placement suitable for stimulators with at least 4 outlets (8 electrode pads) (Figs. 4.22 and 4.23 and Tables 4.19 and 4.20).

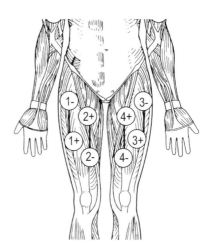

Fig. 4.22 Quadriceps pad layout

Fig. 4.23 Abductors and adductors pad layout

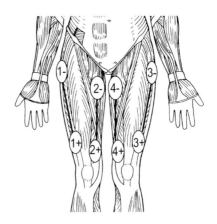

Table 4.19 Quadriceps stimulation parameters female – total time 30 minutes

Phase	1	2	3	4	5	6	7
Time in minutes	5	2	7	5	5	4	2
Stimulation in seconds	4	3	8	3	4	8	2
Pause in seconds	3	2	4	3	3.5	3	0.5
Frequency (Hz)	65	85	10	50	40	10	100
Pulse width in microseconds	340	300	460	300	300	400	80
Ramp in seconds	0.5	0.5	0.5	0.5	0.5	0.5	0.2

Table 4.20 Quadriceps stimulation parameters male – total time 30 minutes

Phase	1	2	3	4	5	6	7
Time in minutes	5	2	7	5	5	4	2
Stimulation in seconds	5	3	8	4	5	8	2
Pause in seconds	4	2	4	3	3.5	3	0.5
Frequency (Hz)	60	70	10	50	40	10	100
Pulse width in microseconds	400	400	600	400	300	500	80
Ramp in seconds	0.5	0.5	0.5	0.5	0.5	0.5	0.2

4.6.3 Gluteus and Hamstrings Stimulation

Phase 1 – preparation: Turn up the stimulation gradually, until an intermittent tingling is felt, then increase the intensity until a gentle pumping is felt.

Phases 2 to 6 – activation: Increase the intensity until a very strong, smooth, visible movement is seen and felt.

Phase 7 – cool down: Turn down the intensity gradually until a mild tingling pulse is felt. Pad placement suitable for stimulators with at least 4 outlets (8 electrode pads) (Figs. 4.24 and 4.25 and Tables 4.21 and 4.22).

Pad placement suitable for stimulators with at least 6 outlets (12 electrode pads). For stimulators with fewer outlets split the stimulation into different sessions, grouping 2 pairs of pad layouts and repeating the stimulation for areas that need the exercise.

Table 4.23 Pectorals, biceps & triceps stimulation parameters female – total time 30 minutes

Phase	1	2	3	4	5	6	7
Time in minutes	5	5	5	5	5	3	2
Stimulation in seconds	2	4	6	4	6	3.5	2
Pause in seconds	2	3	4	3	1	4	0.5
Frequency (Hz)	75	60	10	50	4	70	100
Pulse width in microseconds	200	240	300	200	360	200	80
Ramp in seconds	0.5	0.5	0.5	0.5	0.5	0.5	0.2

Table 4.24 Pectorals, biceps & triceps stimulation parameters male – total time 30 minutes

Phase	1	2	3	4	5	6	7
Time in minutes	5	5	5	5	5	3	2
Stimulation in seconds	2	4	6	4	6	3.5	2
Pause in seconds	2	3	4	3	1	4	0.5
Frequency (Hz)	75	60	10	50	4	70	100
Pulse width in microseconds	200	240	300	200	360	200	80
Ramp in seconds	0.5	0.5	0.5	0.5	0.5	0.5	0.2

4.6.5 Gastrocnemius Stimulation

Phase 1 – preparation: Turn up the stimulation gradually, until an intermittent tingling is felt, then increase the intensity until a gentle pumping is felt.

Phases 2 to 6 – activation: Increase the intensity until a smooth, visible movement is seen and felt.

Phase 7 – cool down: Turn down the intensity gradually until a mild tingling pulse is felt. Pad placement suitable for stimulators with at least 2 outlets (4 electrode pads) (Fig. 4.28 and Tables 4.25 and 4.26).

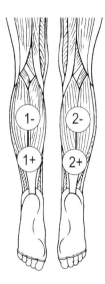

Fig. 4.28 Gastrocnemius pad layout

Table 4.25 Gastrocnemius stimulation parameters female – total time 30 minutes

Phase	1	2	3	4	5	6	7
Time in minutes	5	5	5	5	5	3	2
Stimulation in seconds	4	4	4	4	6	4	2
Pause in seconds	2	3	4	3	1	4	0.5
Frequency (Hz)	10	30	60	50	10	30	100
Pulse width in microseconds	300	240	200	200	360	260	80
Ramp in seconds	0.5	0.5	0.5	0.5	0.5	0.5	0.2

Table 4.26 Gastrocnemius stimulation parameters male – total time 30 minutes

Phase	1	2	3	4	5	6	7
Time in minutes	5	5	5	5	5	3	2
Stimulation in seconds	5	4	4	6	8	4	2
Pause in seconds	3	3	4	3	2	4	0.5
Frequency (Hz)	10	30	65	50	10	30	100
Pulse width in microseconds	360	300	300	300	400	300	80
Ramp in seconds	0.5	0.5	0.5	0.5	0.5	0.5	0.2

4.6.6 Whole Body Stimulation

Phase 1 – preparation: Turn up the stimulation gradually, until an intermittent tingling is felt, then increase the intensity until a gentle pumping is felt.

Phases 2 to 6 – activation: Increase the intensity until a smooth, visible movement is seen and felt.

Phase 7 – cool down: Turn down the intensity gradually until a mild tingling pulse is felt. Pad placement suitable for stimulators with at least 10 outlets (20 electrode pads) (Fig. 4.29 and Tables 4.27 and 4.28).

Table 4.27 Whole body training parameters female – total time 30 minutes

Phase	1	2	3	4	5	6	7
Time in minutes	5	5	5	5	5	3	2
Stimulation in seconds	4	1	4	10	3	6	2
Pause in seconds	4	0.5	4	3	3	4	0.5
Frequency (Hz)	10	80	60	4	40	4	100
Pulse width in microseconds	400	200	200	400	260	400	80
Ramp in seconds	0.5	0.5	0.5	0.5	0.5	0.5	0.2

Table 4.28 Whole body training parameters male – total time 30 minutes

Phase	1	2	3	4	5	6	7
Time in minutes	5	5	5	5	5	3	2
Stimulation in seconds	4	1	5	10	4	6	2
Pause in seconds	4	0.5	4	3	4	4	0.5
Frequency (Hz)	20	70	60	4	40	4	100
Pulse width in microseconds	460	240	220	400	280	400	80
Ramp in seconds	0.5	0.5	0.5	0.5	0.5	0.5	0.2

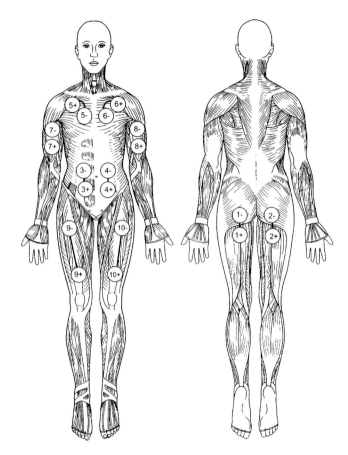

Fig. 4.29 Whole body training pad layout

4.7   Increasing Range of Motion

The following protocols give parameters and pad positioning for people who have had injuries or illnesses which have reduced their range of motion.[35–38] Electrical stimulation can help restore or improve movement capacity with minimum stress, strain or pain. It also lessens weight on load bearing joints as the stimulation treatment is usually given in a reclining or resting position.

The protocols below (Tables 4.29 and 4.30) are suitable for patients who have no permanent nerve damage.

For patients with nerve damage leading to paralysis, the pulse width and stimulation time may need to be dramatically increased in order to elicit a movement. The precise amount of pulse width increase and stimulation time increase will depend on the individual response and should be established by the medical practitioner.

Table 4.29 Range of motion stimulation parameters female – total time 30 minutes

Phase	1	2	3	4	5	6	7
Time in minutes	5	5	5	5	5	3	2
Stimulation in seconds	3	6	2	10	4	4	1.5
Pause in seconds	3.5	5	2.5	3	4.5	4	0.5
Frequency (Hz)	50	10	70	4	35	65	6
Pulse width in microseconds	200	300	200	320	250	200	100
Ramp in seconds	0.5	0.5	0.3	1.3	0.6	0.5	0.2

Table 4.30 Range of motion stimulation parameters male – total time 30 minutes

Phase	1	2	3	4	5	6	7
Time in minutes	5	5	5	5	5	3	2
Stimulation in seconds	3	6	2	10	4	4	1.5
Pause in seconds	3.5	5	2.5	3	4.5	4	0.5
Frequency (Hz)	50	10	70	4	35	65	6
Pulse width in microseconds	200	300	200	320	250	200	100
Ramp in seconds	0.5	0.5	0.3	1.3	0.6	0.5	0.2

Electrode pad positions: the diagrams that follow (Figs. 4.30 to 4.32) show the approximate pad positioning for the various movements. It is essential to experiment somewhat with a light shift in electrode position until a smooth an comfortable movement is obtained as each patient will have a slightly different motor point trigger location. Once the correct electrode pad placement is found, it is advisable to take a photograph of the position so that it can be easily duplicated for further treatment sessions.

The intensity of stimulation for each pair of electrodes also needs to be monitored very closely by the treating practitioner who will decide what sensation and muscular movement is best according to the requirement of the patient.

1. Ankle dorsiflexion
2. Plantar flexion
3. Knee flexion
4. Knee extension
5. Shoulder abduction
6. Hip abduction
7. Finger flexion
8. Finger flexion with wrist flexion
9. Wrist extension
10. Wrist extension and finger extension
11. Elbow extension.

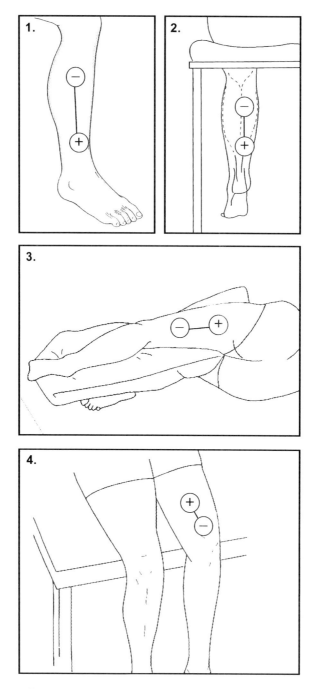

Fig. 4.30 Range of motion 1 – 4 pad layout

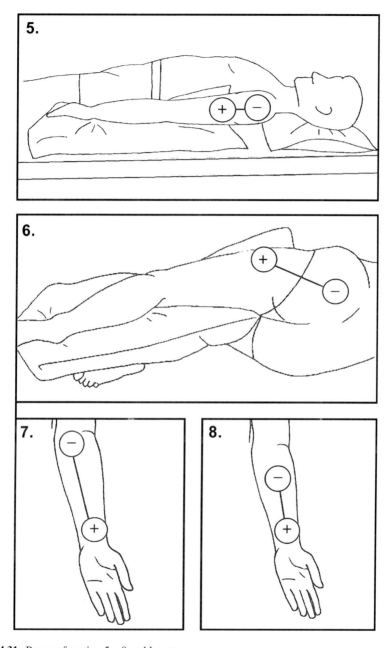

Fig. 4.31 Range of motion 5 – 8 pad layout

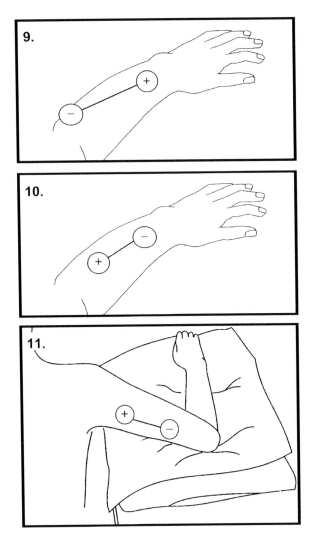

Fig. 4.32 Range of motion 9 – 11 pad layout

4.8   TENS – Transcutaneous Electrical Nerve Stimulation

TENS has now become synonymous with the use of electrical stimulation for pain relief[38–48] and commercially available machines are indeed sold as "TENS" units. This can be quite confusing if one examines the term "transcutaneous electrical nerve stimulation", as most stimulators used for muscle toning, strengthening and body shaping will also stimulate the nerves.

The important issue is to know what parameters are used to attenuate or mask pain and to ensure that the stimulator in question can deliver these signals.

As a general guideline, most commercially available "TENS" units use a weak signal as little intensity is necessary to impede or attenuate pain. This means that very small battery operated machines can be extremely effective if the correct sequence of signals is pre-programmed or made available.

The following protocols list some empirically tested TENS parameters along with the latest consensus regarding the way an electrical signal can attenuate or mask pain.

4.8.1   High TENS – Gate TENS

The gate-control theory suggests that there is a neural mechanism in the spinal cord that acts as a kind of gate, shutting down or opening up the flow of signals from the periphery to the brain. Whether the gate is open, closed or partially closed depends on what sort of signal it receives from the brain to change the perception of pain in the user's body.

These frequencies interfere with the transmission of pain messages at the spinal cord level, and help block their transmission to the brain. Generally, gate TENS parameters are between 75 and 150 Hz (pulse per second) with a narrow pulse width (50–150 microseconds).[49]

4.8.2   Low TENS – Endorphin TENS

Another theory is called 'Endorphin Release', which suggests that electrical impulses stimulate the production of endorphins and enkephalins in the body, the natural morphine-like substances that block pain messages from reaching the brain. An endorphin release TENS has a slow acting effect. The stimulation is applied at a low repetition (pulse) rate between 2 and 10 Hz (pulses per second). Endorphin release type stimulation requires a longer application time, between 30 minutes to 2 hours, to reach a maximum level of endorphin release, but because endorphins remain at effective levels in the blood stream for extended periods, a pain relief period of up to 36 hours may be achieved. Sustained stimulation at low levels of pulse intensity has the strongest effect on managing chronic nagging pain.[49]

The following protocols have varied stimulation parameters for optimum effect and may be used on all the following electrode pad layout positions (Tables 4.31 and 4.32).

Turn up the intensity until the very mildest tingling is felt.

Turn up the intensity until the very mildest tingling is felt. For longer sessions rotate the parameters as above.

Table 4.31 High TENS – Gate TENS stimulation parameters – male & female – total time 30 minutes

Phase	1	2	3	4	5	6	7
Time in minutes	5	3	1	5	3	1	2
Stimulation in seconds	10	3	1	10	3	1	1.2
Pause in seconds	1	4	6	1	4	4	0.5
Frequency (Hz)	100	80	70	100	80	70	100
Pulse width in microseconds	90	90	90	90	90	90	90
Ramp in seconds	0.5	0.5	0.5	0.5	0.5	0.5	0.2

Table 4.32 Low TENS – Endorphin TENS stimulation parameters – male & female – total time 30 minutes–2 hours

Phase	1	2	3	4	5	6	7
Time in minutes	5	3	1	5	3	1	2
Stimulation in seconds	4	10	4	4	10	4	1.2
Pause in seconds	2	1	2	2	1	2	0.5
Frequency (Hz)	4	6	10	4	6	10	2
Pulse width in microseconds	120	120	120	120	120	120	90
Ramp in seconds	0.5	0.5	0.5	0.5	0.5	0.5	0.2

4.9   Repair, Recovery and Rehabilitation

The following suggested protocols and parameters are for general repair, recovery and rehabilitation when there has been a recent injury or when a gentle exercise pattern is indicated (see Figs. 4.33–4.43 and Tables 4.33–4.39).

Turn up the stimulation gradually, until a gentle pulsed tingling is felt. There should be no movement.

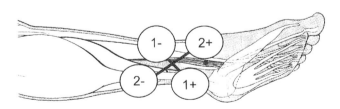

Fig. 4.33 Ankle repair pad layout

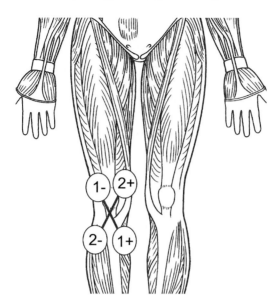

Fig. 4.34 Knee repair pad layout

Table 4.33 Ankle & knee joint stimulation parameters – male & female – total time 20 minutes

Phase	1	2	3	4	5	6	7
Time in minutes	3	3	3	3	3	3	2
Stimulation in seconds	2	4	8	20	6	4	1.2
Pause in seconds	2.5	4	6	1	4	4	0.5
Frequency (Hz)	90	4	10	4	30	65	100
Pulse width in microseconds	100	300	280	300	360	100	100
Ramp in seconds	0.5	0.5	0.5	0.5	0.5	0.5	0.2

Table 4.34 Calf & thigh stimulation parameters – male & female – total time 30 minutes

Phase	1	2	3	4	5	6	7
Time in minutes	5	5	5	5	5	3	2
Stimulation in seconds	2	4	4	3	6	4	3
Pause in seconds	2.5	4	4.5	2	2	4.5	0.5
Frequency (Hz)	10	30	50	60	4	40	75
Pulse width in microseconds	300	250	200	200	400	200	90
Ramp in seconds	0.5	0.5	0.5	0.5	0.7	0.5	0.2

Phase 1 – preparation: Turn up the stimulation gradually, until a gentle pulsed tingling is felt.

Phases 2 to 6 – activation: Increase the intensity until a smooth tensing is felt.

Phase 7 – cool down: Turn down the intensity gradually until a mild tingling pulse is felt. Pad placement suitable for stimulators with at least 2 outlets (4 electrode pads).

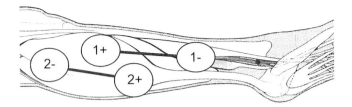

Fig. 4.35 Calf recovery & rehabilitation pad layout

Table 4.35 Inner & outer knee stimulation parameters – male & female – total time 30 minutes

Phase	1	2	3	4	5	6	7
Time in minutes	5	5	5	5	5	3	2
Stimulation in seconds	2	4	4	6	6	4	3
Pause in seconds	2.5	4	4.5	2	2	4.5	0.5
Frequency (Hz)	10	30	50	10	4	40	75
Pulse width in microseconds	200	150	100	100	220	150	90
Ramp in seconds	0.5	0.5	0.5	0.5	0.5	0.5	0.2

Phase 1 – preparation: Turn up the stimulation gradually, until a gentle pulsed tingling is felt.

Phases 2 to 6 – activation: Increase the intensity until a smooth tensing is felt. There should be no movement.

Phase 7 – cool down: Turn down the intensity gradually until a mild tingling pulse is felt. Pad placement suitable for stimulators with at least 2 outlets (4 electrode pads).

The Pad placement below shows the position for either an inner knee ligament injury or an outer knee ligament injury. Select the appropriate layout and place on the injured limb accordingly.

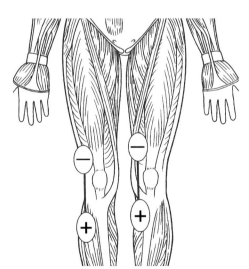

Fig. 4.36 Inner & outer knee ligament repair & recovery pad layout

Table 4.36 Quadriceps recovery & rehabilitation stimulation parameters – male & female – total time 30 minutes

Phase	1	2	3	4	5	6	7
Time in minutes	5	5	5	5	5	3	2
Stimulation in seconds	2	4	4	6	8	4	3
Pause in seconds	2.5	4	4.5	2	2	4.5	0.5
Frequency (Hz)	10	30	50	10	4	40	75
Pulse width in microseconds	200	150	100	100	220	150	90
Ramp in seconds	0.5	0.5	0.5	0.5	0.9	0.5	0.2

Phase 1 – preparation: Turn up the stimulation gradually, until a gentle pulsed tingling is felt.

Phases 2 to 6 – activation: Increase the intensity until a smooth tensing is felt. There should be a gentle balanced movement on both legs. After three sessions, gradually increase the stimulation until a vigorous but comfortable tensing and movement is seen and felt.

Phase 7 – cool down: Turn down the intensity gradually until a mild tingling pulse is felt. Pad placement suitable for stimulators with at least 3 outlets (6 electrode pads).

The Pad placement below shows the position for recovery of an injured right limb. If the injury has occurred on the left limb, simply inverse the pads.

Note: it is always advisable to also stimulate the non injured limb for muscular balance.

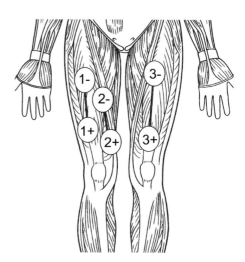

Fig. 4.37 Quadriceps repair & recovery pad layout

Table 4.37 Gluteus & hamstring recovery & rehabilitation stimulation parameters – male & female – total time 30 minutes

Phase	1	2	3	4	5	6	7
Time in minutes	5	5	5	5	5	3	2
Stimulation in seconds	3	4	6	2	8	4	1.5
Pause in seconds	3.5	4	4	2	2	4.5	0.5
Frequency (Hz)	50	30	10	40	4	40	75
Pulse width in microseconds	250	30	400	200	400	200	90
Ramp in seconds	0.5	0.5	0.5	0.5	0.9	0.5	0.2

Phase 1 – preparation: Turn up the stimulation gradually, until a gentle pulsed tingling is felt.

Phases 2 to 6 – activation: Increase the intensity until a smooth tensing is felt. After three sessions, gradually increase the stimulation until a vigorous but comfortable tensing and movement is seen and felt.

Phase 7 – cool down: Turn down the intensity gradually until a mild tingling pulse is felt. Pad placement suitable for stimulators with at least 2 outlets (4 electrode pads).

The Pad placement below shows the position for recovery of an injured right limb. If the injury has occurred on the left limb, simply inverse the pads.

Note: it is always advisable to also stimulate the non injured limb for muscular balance.

After three sessions pad up both sides (suitable for stimulators with 4 outlets).

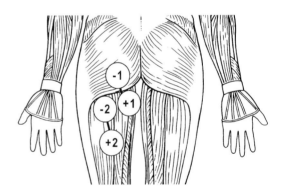

Fig. 4.38 Gluteus & hamstring repair & recovery pad layout

Table 4.38 Hips & Lower back recovery & rehabilitation stimulation parameters – male & female – total time 30 minutes

Phase	1	2	3	4	5	6	7
Time in minutes	5	5	5	5	5	3	2
Stimulation in seconds	3	4	6	2	8	4	1.5
Pause in seconds	3.5	4	4	2	2	4.5	0.5
Frequency (Hz)	10	30	4	50	4	30	75
Pulse width in microseconds	250	250	300	200	350	200	90
Ramp in seconds	0.5	0.5	0.5	0.5	0.9	0.5	0.2

Phase 1 – preparation: Turn up the stimulation gradually, until a gentle pulsed tingling is felt.

Phases 2 to 6 – activation: Increase the intensity until a smooth tensing is felt. No movement should be seen.

Phase 7 – cool down: Turn down the intensity gradually until a mild tingling pulse is felt. Pad placement suitable for stimulators with at least 4 outlets (8 electrode pads).

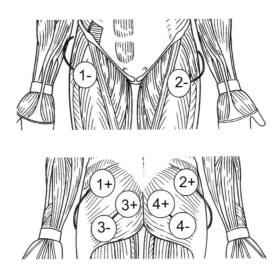

Fig. 4.39 Hips repair & recovery pad layout

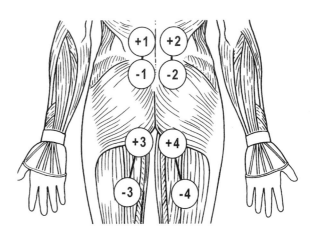

Fig. 4.40 Lower back, gluteus & hamstring repair & recovery pad layout

Fig. 4.41 Lower back repair & recovery pad layout

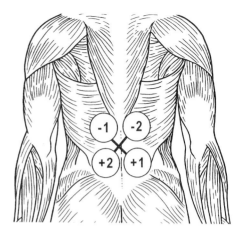

Table 4.39 Middle & back recovery & rehabilitation stimulation parameters – male & female – total time 30 minutes

Phase	1	2	3	4	5	6	7
Time in minutes	5	5	5	5	5	3	2
Stimulation in seconds	1.5	4	2	2	5	4	1.5
Pause in seconds	0.5	4	2.5	2	5	4.5	0.5
Frequency (Hz)	80	4	20	10	4	30	75
Pulse width in microseconds	150	250	200	220	250	150	90
Ramp in seconds	0.2	0.5	0.5	0.5	0.5	0.5	0.2

Phase 1 – preparation: Turn up the stimulation gradually, until a gentle pulsed tingling is felt.

Phases 2 to 6 – activation: Increase the intensity until a very gentle tensing is felt. No movement should be seen.

Phase 7 – cool down: Turn down the intensity gradually until a mild tingling pulse is felt. Pad placement suitable for stimulators with at least 4 outlets (8 electrode pads).

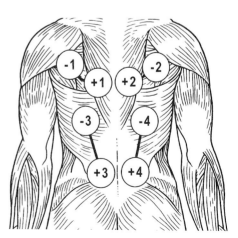

Fig. 4.42 Lower & middle back repair & recovery pad layout

Fig. 4.43 Upper back repair & recovery pad layout

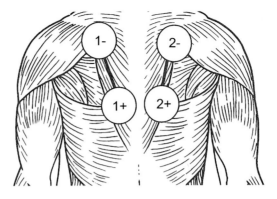

4.9.1 RSI – Repetitive Strain Injury

Often a repeated movement may lead to pain and strain of muscle, tendon and joint. Electrical stimulation has been used as a very effective pain relief and recovery tool for this condition and can also act as a preventative treatment. The following protocols for recovery and rehabilitation, may also be used to treat RSI (see Figs. 4.44–4.48 and Tables 4.40–4.43).

Table 4.40 Shoulders RSI, recovery & rehabilitation stimulation parameters – male & female – total time 30 minutes

Phase	1	2	3	4	5	6	7
Time in minutes	5	5	5	5	5	3	2
Stimulation in seconds	4	8	2	5	4	8	1.5
Pause in seconds	4	2	2.5	3	4.5	4	0.5
Frequency (Hz)	10	4	30	10	50	4	75
Pulse width in microseconds	300	300	200	300	150	300	90
Ramp in seconds	0.2	0.5	0.5	0.5	0.5	0.5	0.2

Phase 1 – preparation: Turn up the stimulation gradually, until a gentle pulsed tingling is felt.

Phases 2 to 6 – activation: Increase the intensity until a very gentle tensing is felt. A faint movement might be seen.

Phase 7 – cool down: Turn down the intensity gradually until a mild tingling pulse is felt. Pad placement suitable for stimulators with at least 4 outlets (8 electrode pads).

Turn up the stimulation gradually, until a gentle pulsed tingling is felt. There should be no movement.

Fig. 4.44 Shoulders RSI, repair & recovery pad layout

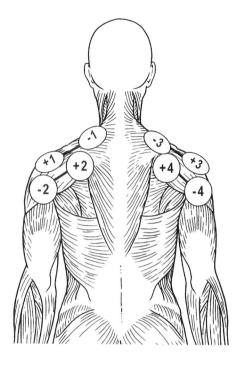

Table 4.41 Elbow RSI, recovery & rehabilitation stimulation parameters – male & female – total time 30 minutes

Phase	1	2	3	4	5	6	7
Time in minutes	5	5	5	5	5	3	2
Stimulation in seconds	4	6	2	3	4	8	1.5
Pause in seconds	2	2	2.5	3	4.5	4	0.5
Frequency (Hz)	80	4	30	10	20	4	75
Pulse width in microseconds	100	300	150	200	200	300	90
Ramp in seconds	0.2	0.5	0.5	0.5	0.5	0.5	0.2

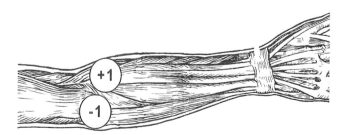

Fig. 4.45 Elbow RSI, repair & recovery pad layout

Table 4.42 Wrist flexion RSI, recovery & rehabilitation stimulation parameters – male & female – total time 30 minutes

Phase	1	2	3	4	5	6	7
Time in minutes	5	5	5	5	5	3	2
Stimulation in seconds	4	8	2	5	4	8	1.5
Pause in seconds	4	2	2.5	3	4.5	4	0.5
Frequency (Hz)	10	4	30	10	50	4	75
Pulse width in microseconds	300	300	200	300	150	300	90
Ramp in seconds	0.2	0.5	0.5	0.5	0.5	0.5	0.2

Phase 1 – preparation: Turn up the stimulation gradually, until a gentle pulsed tingling is felt.

Phases 2 to 6 – activation: Increase the intensity until a very gentle tensing is felt. A faint flexing of the wrist should be seen.

Phase 7 – cool down: Turn down the intensity gradually until a mild tingling pulse is felt. Pad placement suitable for stimulators with 1 outlet (2 electrode pads).

Alternate this pad placement (Fig. 4.46) and protocol with the wrist repair one that follows (Fig. 4.47).

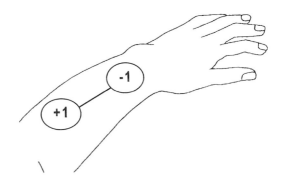

Fig. 4.46 Wrist flexion RSI, repair & recovery pad layout

Table 4.43 Wrist & hand repair stimulation parameters – male & female – total time 30 minutes

Phase	1	2	3	4	5	6	7
Time in minutes	5	5	5	5	5	3	2
Stimulation in seconds	4	8	2	5	4	8	1.5
Pause in seconds	4	2	2.5	3	4.5	4	0.5
Frequency (Hz)	10	4	30	10	50	4	75
Pulse width in microseconds	300	300	200	300	150	300	90
Ramp in seconds	0.2	0.5	0.5	0.5	0.5	0.5	0.2

Turn up the stimulation gradually, until a gentle pulsed tingling is felt. Pad placement suitable for stimulators with 2 outlet (4 electrode pads).

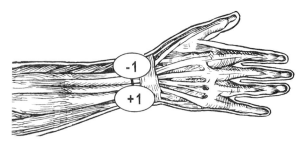

Fig. 4.47 Wrist repair pad layout

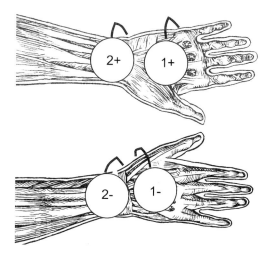

Fig. 4.48 Wrist & hand circulation & repair pad layout

Acknowledgement   I would like to thank my father, Herman Schaefer, pioneer of electrical stimulation, and Professors Gerta Vrbová and Olga Hudlicka, for enhancing my knowledge of the subject. I would also like to thank Ultratone for the use of their copyrighted figures in this chapter.

References

1. Herman Schaefer founded Slendertone Ltd in 1964, Companies House London No 00838231, later incorporated as part of Ultratone Scientific Instruments Ltd. (No. 01432229, 1989).
2. J. P. Porcari, J. Miller, K. Cornwell, C. Foster, M. Gibson, K. McLean, and T. Kernozek, The effects of neuromuscular stimulation training on abdominal strength, endurance and selected anthropometric measure, *J. Sports Sci. Med.* **4**:66–75 (2005).
3. E. Ballantine, and B. Donne, Effects of neuromuscular electrical stimulation on static and dynamic abdominal strength and endurance in healthy males, 4th Annual Congress of the European College of Sports Science, Rome, 14–17 July 1999.

4. G. Alon, S. A. McCombe, S. Koutsantinis, L. J. Stumphauzer, K. C. Burgwin, M. M. Parent, and R. A. Bosworth, Comparison of the effects of electrical stimulation and exercise on abdominal musculature, *J. Orthopaed. Sports Phy. Therap.* **8**:567–573 (1987).

5. N. Babault, G. Cometti, M. Bernardin, M. Pousson, and J. C. Chatard, Effects of electromyostimulation training on muscle strength and power of elite rugby players. *J. Strength Cond. Res.* **21**: 431–437 (2007).

6. J. F. Hopp, and W. K. Palmer, Effect of electrical stimulation on intracellular triacylglycerol in isolated skeletal muscle, *J. Appl. Physiol.* **68**:348–354 (1990).

7. J. F. Hopp, and W. K. Palmer, Electrical stimulation alters fatty acid metabolism in isolated skeletal muscle, *J. Appl. Physiol.* **68**:2473–2481 (1990).

8. G. Pedini, and P. Zaietta, On some aspects of activation of tissue lipolysis by electric factors, *Minerva Med.* **66**:324–329 (1975).

9. M. Ruffin, and S. Micolaidis, Electrical stimulation of the ventromedial hypothalamus enhances both fat utilization and metabolic rate that precede and parallel the inhibition of feeding behaviour, *Brain Res.* **846**:23–29 (1999).

10. P. Banerjee, B. Caulfield, L. Crowe, and A. Clark, Prolonged electrical muscle stimulation exercise improves strength and aerobic capacity in healthy sedentary adults, *J. Appl. Physiol.* **99**:2307–2311 (2005).

11. D. Pette, and G. Vrbová, What does chronic electrical stimulation teach us about muscle plasticity? *Muscle Nerve* **22**:666–677 (1999).

12. A. J. Robinson, and L. Snyder-Mackler, *Clinical Electrophysiology* (Williams & Wilkins, Baltimore, 1992).

13. V. Dubowitz, S. A. Hyde, O. Scott, and G. Vrbová, Effect of long term electrical stimulation on the fatigue of human muscle, Presented at the Physiological Society Annual Conference, UCL, London, March 26,27, 1982.

14. G. Vrbová, Considerations for the therapeutic use of chronic electrical stimulation of skeletal muscles, Newsletter of the Department of Anatomy and Embryology, University College London, March 1982.

15. G. M. Eom, T. Watanabe, N. Hoshimiya, and G. Khang, Gradual potentiation of isometric muscle force during constant electrical stimulation, *Med. Biol. Eng. Comput.* **40**:137–143 (2002).

16. P. Chan, and K. I. Kwann, The frequency-specificity theory, *Hong Kong Physiother. J.* **13**:23–27 (1991/1992).

17. I. O. W. Man, G. S. Lepar, M. C. Morrissey, and J. K. Cywinski, Effect of neuromuscular electrical stimulation on foot and ankle volume during standing. *Med. Sci. Sports Exerc.* **35**:630–634 (2003).

18. J. Kahn, *Principles and Practices of Electrotherapy* (Churchill Livingstone, New York, 1994).

19. J. Low, and A. Reed, *Electrotherapy Explained* (Butterworth & Heinman, Oxford, 1994).

20. H. X. Liu, J. B. Tian, F. Luo, Y. H. Jiang, Z. G. Deng, L. Xiong, C. Liu, J. S. Wang, and J. S. Han, Repeated 100 Hz TENS for the treatment of chronic inflammatory hyperalgesia and suppression of spinal release of substance P in monoarthritic rats. *Evid. Based Complement. Alternat. Med.* **4**:65–75 (2007).

21. O. Scott, S. Kitchen, and S. Bazin, *Clayton's Electrotherapy* (W.B. Saunders, London, 1998).

22. D. Poole, Use of tens in pain management. Part One: How TENS works, *Nurs. Times* **103**:28–29 (2007).

23. M. Erdogan, A. Erdogan, N. Erbil, H. K. Karakaya, and A. Demircan, Prospective, randomized, placebo-controlled study of the effect of TENS on postthoracotomy pain and pulmonary function, *World J. Surg.* **29**:1563–1570 (2005).

24. T. Nalty, *Electrotherapy Clinical Procedures Manual* (McGraw-Hill, New York, 2001).

25. H. Waldorf, and J. Fewkes, Wound healing, *Adv. Dermatol.* **10**:77–97 (1995).

26. E. M. Wojtys, J. E. Carpenter, and G. A. Ott, Electrical stimulation of soft tissues, *Instr. Course Lect.* **42**:443–452 (1993).

27. M. T. Omar, A. M. El-Badawy, W. H. Borhan, and A. A. Nossier, Improvement of oedema and hand function in superficial and second degree hand burns using electrical stimulation, *Egypt J. Plast. Reconstr. Surg.* **28**:141–147 (2004).

28. E. M. Wojtys, J. E. Carpenter, and G. A. Ott, Electrical stimulation of soft tissues, *Instr. Course Lect.* **42**:443–452 (1993).

29. G. D. Gentzkow, Electrical stimulation to heal dermal wounds, *J. Dermatol. Surg. Oncol.* **19**:753–758 (1993).

30. J. A. Feedar, L. C. Kloth, and G. D. Gentzkow, Chronic dermal ulcer healing enhanced with monophasic pulsed electrical stimulation, *Phys. Ther.* **71**:639–649 (1991).

31. W. D. Currier, Effects of electronic stimulation of the VII nerve. On senescent changes of the face, Ann. Otol. Rhinol. Laryngol. **72:**289–306 (1963).

32. A. A. Al-Majed, C. M. Neumann, T. M. Brushart, and T. Gordon, Brief electrical stimulation promotes the speed and accuracy of motor axonal regeneration, *J. Neurosci.* **20**:2602–2608 (2000).

33. M. S. Agren, M. A. Engel, and P. M. Mertz, Collagenase during burn wound healing: influence of a hydrogel dressing and pulsed electrical stimulation, *Plast. Reconstr. Surg.* **94**:518–524 (1994).

34. F. Bobanović, S. Simči, V. Kotnik, and L. Vodovnik, Pulsed electrical current enhances the phorbol ester induced oxidative burst in human neutrophils, *FEBS Lett.* **311**:95–98 (1992).

35. Y. N. Berner, O. Lif Kimchi, V. Spokoiny, and B. Finkeltov, The effect of electric stimulation treatment on the functional rehabilitation of acute geriatric patients with stroke – a preliminary study. *Arch. Gerontol. Geriatr.* **39**:125–132 (2004).

36. S. N. Kukke, and R. J. Triolo, The effects of trunk stimulation on bimanual seated workspace. *IEEE Trans. Neural. Syst. Rehabil. Eng.* **12**:177–185 (2004).

37. W. D. Memberg, P. E. Crago, and M. W. Keith, Restoration of elbow extension via functional electrical stimulation in individuals with tetraplegia. *J. Rehabil. Res. Dev.* **40**:477–486 (2003).

38. T. Yanagi, N. Shiba, T. Maeda, K. Iwasa, Y. Umezu, Y. Tagawa, S. Matsuo, K. Nagata, T. Yamamoto, and J. R. Basford, Agonist contractions against electrically stimulated antagonists. *Arch. Phys. Med. Rehabil.* **84**:843–848 (2003).

39. D. N. Rushton, Electrical stimulation in the treatment of pain. *Disabil. Rehabil.* **24**:407–515 (2002).

40. M. M. Ng, M. C. Leung, and D. M. Poon, The effects of electro-acupuncture and transcutaneous electrical nerve stimulation on patients with painful osteoarthritic knees: a randomised controlled trial with follow-up evaluation. *J. Alternat. Complement. Med.* **9**:641–649 (2003).

41. L. S. Chesterton, N. E. Foster, C. C. Wright, G. D. Baxter, and P. Barlas, Effects of TENS frequency, intensity and stimulation site parameter manipulation on pressure pain thresholds in healthy human subjects. *Pain* **106**:73–80 (2003).

42. M. Osiri, V. Welch, L. Brosseau, B. Shea, J. McGowan, P. Tugwell, and G. Wells, Transcutaneous electrical nerve stimulation for knee osteoarthritis. *Cochrane Database Systematic Reviews* **4**:CD002823 (2000).

43. W. P. Cooney, Electrical stimulation and the treatment of complex regional pain syndromes of the upper extremity. *Hand Clin.* **13**:519–526 (1997).

44. T. Forst, M. Nguyen, S. Forst, B. Disselhoff, T. Pohlmann, and A. Pfutzner, Impact of low frequency transcutaneous electrical nerve stimulation on symptomatic diabetic neuropathy using the new Salutaris device. *Diabetes Nutr. Metab.* **17**:163–168 (2004).

45. A. Kararmaz, S. Kaya, H. Karaman, and S. Turhanoglu, Effect of the frequency of transcutaneous electrical nerve stimulation on analgesia during extracorporeal shock wave lithotripsy. *Urol. Res.* **32**:411–415 (2004).

46. L. S. Chesterton, P. Barlas, N. E. Foster, G. D. Baxter, and C. C. Wright, Gender differences in pressure pain threshold in healthy humans. *Pain* **101**:259–266 (2003).

47. G. L. Cheing, A. Y. Tsui, S. K. Lo, and C. W. Hui-Chan, Optimal stimulation duration of tens in the management of osteoarthritic knee pain. *J. Rehabil. Med.* **35**:62–68 (2003).

48. J. T. van der Spank, D. C. Cambier, H. M. De Paepe, L. A. Danneels, E. E. Witvrouw, and L. Beerens, Pain relief in labour by transcutaneous electrical nerve stimulation (TENS). *Arch. Gynecol. Obstet.* **264**:131–136 (2000).

49. J. Kahn, *Principles and Practice of Electrotherapy* (Churchill Livingstone, New York, 1987).

Index

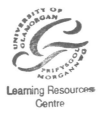